FOREW(

Originally published in 1895 by t
House," Ulrico Hoepli Publisher in
Poisonings" is a valuable work not only or not so much for the
study of toxicology, but for its role as an important historical and
social testimony.

While some notions reported by Dr. Ferraris are still valid, most
have been integrated, improved, or even surpassed over time.
Yet, the reading is interesting and smooth, able to effectively
transport us back to a lost time, where we seem to see Dr. Jekyll at
work with his potions, Cesare Lombroso with his physiognomic
measurements, and in another chapter, Sherlock Holmes
searching for clues of poisoning, while Jack "The Ripper" is,
nocturnally, hunting his next victim.

The text discusses the different types of poison (caustic, irritating,
exciting, paralyzing, and of the blood), the symptoms of poisoning,
and possible remedies. It also covers those intoxicating substances
that are taken voluntarily, like alcohol, hemp, cocaine, and ether
– the drinkers of which "*enjoy good health*", but Dr. Ferraris notes:
"*It has long been and universally recognized that the use of such an
intoxicant shortens life*". Enjoy your reading.

Turin, November 2023

C.R.

POISONS AND POISONINGS

Dr. COSTANTE FERRARIS

POISONS
AND
POISONINGS

WITH 20 ENGRAVINGS

First Edition 1895

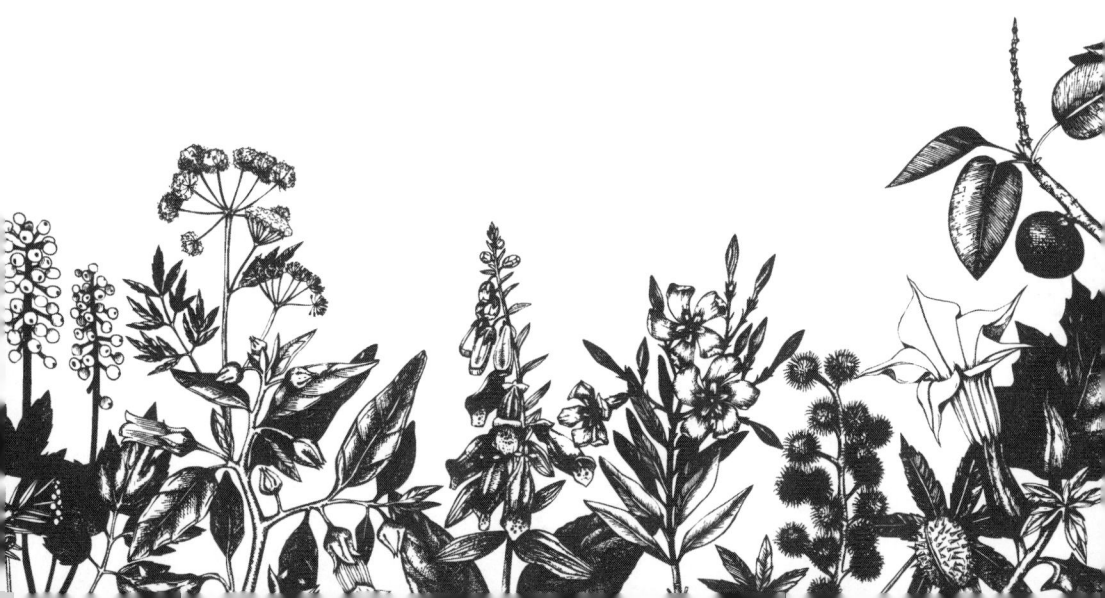

INDEX

Caustic Poisons.

Irritant Poisons.

Excitant Poisons.

Paralyzing Poisons.

Blood Poisons.

TO THE READER

The title of this book sufficiently indicates its nature and purpose, thus sparing me from writing the preface, and above all saving you the boredom of reading it; allow me just a brief declaration.

In embarking on this work, I set myself the goal of compiling a practical manual that in a few pages, with the greatest possible brevity and clarity, summarizes the main physical and chemical characteristics of toxic substances, the most important symptoms, the most characteristic anatomical alterations caused by their absorption by the organism, the most effective drugs to mitigate or neutralize their harmful action, a book that, in a word, provides the reader with the indispensable elements for the diagnosis and treatment of poisonings. If self-love does not blind me, I believe I have achieved my intention; certainly, I have not neglected any of the means at my disposal for this purpose, and I hope in any case that my work, though modest and imperfect, will not be entirely useless nor devoid of merits.

Turin, October 1896

Dr. C. FERRARIS

BIBLIOGRAPHY

WORKS.

M. Orfila: *Traité de toxicologie*. Paris, Labé, éd., 1852 - C.P. Galtier: *Traité de toxicologie*. Paris, Chamerot, éd., 1855- M. Bouchardat: *Manuel de matière médicale, de thérapeutique et de pharmacie*. Paris, Germer Baillière, éd., 1856 - M. Vernois: *Traité pratique d' hygiène industrielle*. Paris, J. B. Baillière et fils, éd., 1860 - A. Tardieu: *Étude médico-légale sur l'empoisonnement*. Id. id. 1867 - A. Cantani: *Manuale di materia medica e terapeutica*. Milano, D. F. Vallardi, ed., 1869 - O. Schmiedeberg u. R. Koppe: *Das muscarin*. Leipzig, 1869 - O. Liebreich: *Das chloralhydrat*. Berlin, 1869 - Dragendorff: *Manuel de toxicologie* traduit por E. Ritter. Paris, F. Savy, éd, 1873 - A. Naquet: *Principes de chimie*. Paris, F. Savy, éd., 1875 - W. Hommond: *Traité des maladies du systéme nerveux*. Traduction française por F. Labadie-Lagrave. Paris, J. B. Baillière et fils, éd., 1879 - H. A. Depierris: *Le tabac*. Paris, E. Dentu, éd., 1876 - M. Semmola: *Manuale di materia medica*. Napoli, D. Cesareo, ed., 1880 - A. S. Taylor: *Traité de médecine légale,* traduit sur la dixième édition anglaise par Henry Coutagne. Puris, Germer Baillière etc.[ie], éd., 1881 - A. Vulpian: *Leçons sur l'action physiologique des substances toxiques et medicamenteuses.* Paris, O. Doin, éd., 1881-82 - F. A. Falck: *L'Antagonismo dei veleni* (Conferenza tenuta il 18 luglio 1878 nel Circolo Fisiologico di Kiel). Raccolta di conferenze cliniche. Milano, D. L. Vallardi, ed., 1882 - T. Husemann: *Trattato di terapeutica*, versione italiana del Prof. A. Raffaele. Napoli, R. Marghieri, ed., 1883 - H. Baillon: *Traité de botanlque médicale.* Paris, Hachette, éd., 1884 - N. Du Moulin: *La toxicologie du cuivre.* Bruxelles, A. Mancenux, éd., 1886 - C. Hischmann: *Intoxication et hystérie.* Paris, G. Steinheil, éd., 1888 - Vétault Victor: *Étude médico-légale sur l'alcoolisme.* Paris, J. B. Baillière et fils, éd., 1887 - J. Arnould: *Nouveaux éléments d'hygiéne.* Id., id., 1889 - A. Chapuis: *Précis de toxicologie.* Paris, J. B Baillière et fils, éd., 1889 - H. Guimbail: *Le morphinomanes.* Id. id., 1892 - E. Pollacci: *Corso di chimica medico-farmaceutica.* Milano, Fratelli Dumolard, 1892-93 - P. Giacosa: *Trattato di materia medica, farmacologia e tossicologia.* Torino, Frat. Bocca, ed., 1893 - G. Hayem: *Leçons de thérapeutique,* Paris, G. Masson, éd., 1887-90-91-93 - I. Guareschi: *Supplemento annuale all'Enciclopedia di chimica.* Torino, l888-80-93-94-95 - Dujardin-Beaumetz: *Dictionnaire de thérapeutique, de matiére médicale, de pharmacologie, de toxicologie.* Paris, O. Doin, éd., 1890-95.

MAGAZINES.

Annali di chimica e farmacologia. Milano, 1893-94-96 - *Revue médicale.* Louvain, 1891 - *Le progrés médical.* Paris, 1890-91-92 - *Il Policlinico.* Roma, 1894-95 - *Revue des sciences médicales.* Paris, 1894-95 - *Gazzetta degli Ospitali.* Milano, 1892-93-95 - *Berliner Klinische Wochenschrift,* 1895 - *La semaine médicale.* Paris, 1895-96 - *La Riforma medica.* Napoli, 1893-94-95-96.

General Considerations on Poisons and Poisonings

A *poison* is understood to be any solid, liquid, or gaseous substance that, when absorbed by the body, can cause structural alterations or functional disturbances of varying intensity, causing death, or at least putting life in serious danger.

However, the issue is not as simple as it might initially appear, since in practice it is very difficult to draw a clear line between poison and medication. Everything ultimately comes down to the dose at which these substances are administered. Many of them, in high doses, cause horrifying, disastrous effects, yet when given in appropriate quantities, they prove to be highly useful medicines, utilized by therapy to effectively combat a wide range of serious diseases.

It is known that a single drop of prussic acid, falling on a mucous membrane, can cause instantaneous death; this same acid, suitably diluted, becomes a valuable drug. On the other hand, almost all substances used as medicines can, if absorbed in large quantities, act as poisons.

But, in evaluating the toxicity of a given substance, one must also take into account the age of the individual to whom it is administered; the dose that is medicinal for an adult becomes toxic for a child.

Influence of Habit. - The effect of many poisons is diminished by habit. Without going back to historical examples that everyone knows, it will suffice to mention opium eaters and arsenic eaters. These individuals can safely ingest a dose of poison that would certainly be lethal to someone who is not accustomed to it. *Schroff* noted a case of death from just two pipes of tobacco, a dose that is absolutely insignificant for a smoker.

Idiosyncrasy. - With this term, we wish to define the special predisposition of the organism, by virtue of which external agents, whatever their nature, produce different effects than those they usually produce. Thus, many medications, even at therapeutic doses, have toxic effects in certain individuals, while others can tolerate doses that would be lethal for the average person. *Christison* recalls a notable case where a man unaccustomed to opium took 28 grams of laudanum without experiencing any effect. This latter form of idiosyncrasy is extremely rare.

Other influences. - Some diseases give the body a special tolerance for many poisons and medications. Individuals affected by rabies or tetanus can ingest very strong doses of opium without experiencing severe disturbances; the same is observed for antimony preparations in lung diseases.

Taylor speaks of a 29-year-old hemiplegic woman who took a daily dose of three grains of strychnine for six days without unpleasant consequences, while a single grain of strychnine is commonly considered a lethal dose for a healthy adult. Conversely, certain morbid states undoubtedly increase the susceptibility of the organism to certain toxic substances; this fact can be observed for arsenic and antimony or other irritants in individuals suffering from gastroenteritis, for mercury in those suffering from kidney ailments, and for opium in the elderly affected by lung diseases, or who are prone to apoplexy.

Another very important influence is the method of administration of poisons. These can be administered in more or less voluminous fragments, in more or less fine powder, in solution, or even in the form of gas or vapors. Their activity will be maximal, almost instantaneous in the latter case; it will also be high for poisons in solution, low for those in powder, and minimal for those in large fragments.

The same dose of poison will also exert a different action depending on the state of fullness or emptiness of the stomach; stomach fullness can go so far as to completely suspend the absorption of the poison and prevent poisoning. *Hoffmann* speaks of a charlatan to whom 60 centigrams of arsenious acid caused almost no disturbance because he had previously drunk a large amount of milk, which was soon vomited up along with the poison. *Orfila* cites the case of several people who ate a cake at a banquet in which arsenious acid had been placed instead of flour; all the guests who had until then eaten and drunk little died in a short time, while those with full stomachs were saved by vomiting.

Paths of Poison absorption. - For a toxic substance to exert its action on the body, it must be absorbed, i.e., it must mix with the mass of blood that distributes it to various organs. This absorption can occur from the gastroenteric mucosa (ingestion is undoubtedly the most frequent method of administering poisons), or from the mucosa of the respiratory tract, which also has great absorbing power, or even, albeit to a lesser extent, from mucous membranes lined with columnar epithelium (uterus, vagina, urethra, etc.).

The skin, when the epidermis is intact, is very poorly suited for absorption; it is quite different when, for whatever reason, there is even a very superficial flaking of the horny layer. The exposed dermis, the surface of ulcers, sores, and the subcutaneous cellular tissue are also endowed with a very energetic absorbing power. Lastly, poisons can be directly brought into contact with the blood (wounds, venous injections).

Action of Poisons. - Considered in a general way, the action of most poisonous substances is dual and includes a *local* action, which is exerted on the parts with which the poison comes into contact, and a *general* action resulting from its absorption.

The local action predominates only for a small number of poisons. Sometimes it is entirely limited to the point that was struck by the poison, where its effects seem to exhaust themselves; in other cases, the toxin, applied to the surface of the skin or mucous membranes, or injected into the subcutaneous cellular tissue, penetrates by imbibition into nearby organs where it exerts its influence.

The general action of poisons is the consequence and proof of their absorption. It is in the organs to which they are carried by the circulatory stream, and especially in those where the flow is slowing down, such as in the large secretory organs (liver, kidneys), that absorbed poisons can be found much more reliably than at their point of entry, where their rapid passage and partial expulsion would often make it very difficult to trace them. This fact of the absorption of toxic substances is constant and general, even for those where the local action predominates. The most energetic concentrated acids, caustic alkalis, do not limit their action to the burn they produce, but are partially absorbed, exert an obvious action on the blood, and analysis finds their presence in various viscera.

Paths of Elimination. - There are multiple ways through which poisons are eliminated from the body. They can be expelled through the gastrointestinal tract (vomiting, diarrhea); through the respiratory pathways (alcohol, ether, chloroform); through the skin via sweat (mercury); through the mammary glands in milk (iodine); through the salivary glands (mercury); through the liver via bile (lead, zinc); and through the kidneys (Spanish fly, potassium iodide, etc.). Death can occur, however, when the amount of poison introduced exceeds the amount that is eliminated.

Anatomical Lesions. - These can vary greatly, sometimes being minimal or not easily observable. Depending on the way the poison acts, they should be categorized as either local or general, and first sought in the digestive organs and on the parts directly hit by the poison. The second kind should be searched for in all the organs where it was carried by the blood, especially in those that, due to their structure and function, are susceptible to the poison's more prolonged and deeper action. These include the liver, where blood accumulates, and the kidneys, which are the main agents for the elimination of absorbed poisons.

Causes of Poisoning. - In many cases, poison is the *last resort* to which a person contemplating suicide turns to end their own physical or emotional suffering. At other times, it is a weapon used to seriously harm or kill another individual.

Often, poisoning is nothing more than the result of a fatal oversight, a mistake that causes one to confuse a highly potent poison for an innocuous substance. Such is the case with arsenic acid, which was mistaken for wheat flour; or poisonous mushrooms, which are often confused with edible species. Even more common is poisoning for purely indulgent purposes; driven by a compelling need that habit ingrains in the body. Notable examples include opium eaters, morphine addicts, smokers, and alcoholics.

Many professions expose countless individuals to an atmosphere saturated with harmful emissions; occupational poisoning is extremely common among workers handling lead, or those who have to deal daily with arsenic or mercury. Another important cause can be traced back to the neglect of basic kitchen hygiene standards (poorly sealed pots, cookware containing lead, poorly cleaned copper utensils, etc.) or in the living environment (rooms painted with lead-based paint or wallpapered with arsenic-tinted paper, or heated with old, poorly constructed iron stoves, etc.). Everyone knows that bites from certain animals, especially snakes, can lead to severe, often fatal, poisoning, which manifests rapidly due to the direct injection of the venom into the blood. Another cause, as we've said, can be attributed to idiosyncrasy.

Common Symptoms. - In the clinical picture of poisoning, we generally first notice a disturbance in digestive function, followed by more or less severe alterations in circulation and respiration; lastly, there is a primary or secondary disorder of the nervous system. The onset of symptoms is generally rapid, in some cases instantaneous; even with poisonous mushrooms, which can remain in the stomach for 12 or more hours without producing any symptoms. *Peddie* observed poisoning occurring just half an hour after ingestion.

Therapy. - In the treatment of poisonings, the first aim is to remove the poison from the body, an objective that can be achieved through various means. The foremost among these is emptying the stomach, either by administering emetics or by using gastric lavage. For the latter, a hard probe should not be used to avoid damaging parts possibly already corroded by the poison, nor should a gastric pump be used, which could remove pieces of mucosa (*Lewin*). Instead, a rubber tube of 8-10 millimeters in diameter and 2 meters in length should be used, to which a rubber bulb can be attached, functioning as both a suction and pressing device.

These gastric lavages can also be easily performed on individuals who are completely unconscious and should not be neglected even when severe symptoms of absorption have already set in, due to the possibility of eliminating at least the portion of the poison that remains in the stomach. Even if poisoning occurred via subcutaneous injection, or medicinal injections into the pleura or cystic cavities, it is still advisable to empty the stomach because some toxins (like iodine, morphine, etc.) introduced in this manner are eliminated by the gastric mucosa. For lavages, plain water can be used; however, once the nature of the poison is identified, liquids containing the antidote should be used. To combat persistent vomiting due to irritation of the gastric mucosa, a solution of cocaine hydrochloride (0.05 - 0.10:1000) may be useful for the lavages; intense inflammation will be calmed with cold water rinses; and gastric hemorrhages can be stopped with a dilute solution of ferric perchloride.

Emetics are less effective than gastric lavage, as even the most violent vomiting often fails to dislodge poison particles strongly adhering to the stomach's mucosa. Therefore, they should only be used when, for whatever reason, stomach lavage is not possible. In any case, vomiting should not be induced with oily or fatty substances, or by drinking hot water, as this can make many poisons soluble. The best emetics in these cases are a few grams of mustard diluted in a glass of water, copper sulfate (1 gram per 100 of distilled water), or a subcutaneous injection of apomorphine hydrochloride (2 centigrams).

Since, despite quickly performed lavage, many toxic substances can easily pass from the stomach to the intestines, it is important to ensure their elimination through this route by administering laxatives (sodium or magnesium sulfate) dissolved in water, in potion or introduced into the stomach with a probe. At the same time, evacuative enemas will be administered.

The second indication, namely the chemical neutralization of the poison, can generally only be achieved if the poison is still in the stomach. Alkalis will be given for acid poisoning, or conversely acids when the poison is alkaline; hydrated iron peroxide will be injected into the stomach to neutralize arsenic, etc. However, little can be expected from the use of antidotes once the poison has entered the bloodstream unless one can benefit from the action of antagonists (morphine and atropine; pilocarpine and atropine, etc.).

Lastly, as for the means to counter severe functional disturbances due to absorption, they vary according to the symptoms that dominate in each case. Cardiac weakness will be fought with stimulants, which Lewin advises to administer through enemas rather than subcutaneous injections, as the latter often cannot be absorbed due to impaired or arrested peripheral circulation. He recommends liquid ammonia (30 drops in 2 glasses of water), cognac (1 teaspoon per glass of water mixed with a gum solution), and camphorated oil at 10:100 (a teaspoon mixed with a sufficient amount of any oily substance) for such stimulant enemas. If the subcutaneous tissue retains its absorptive capacity, he believes the best stimulant to be musk tincture (3-4 grams per subcutaneous injection). To revive the patient, skin irritants (mustard plasters, etc.) and stimulants will be used. Against convulsions, ether or chloroform inhalations will be used; paralysis of the respiratory centers will be fought with cold compresses on the nape and artificial respiration. Lewin advises against ammonia inhalation, as it can only have an inhibitory effect on already weakened respiratory movements. Finally, in cases of severe blood alteration, generous bloodletting will be performed, followed by an intravenous injection of physiological solution (0.6:100) of sodium chloride, the quantity of which will be about double that of the blood drawn from the phlebotomy.

CAUSTIC POISONS

I. Concentrated Mineral Acids

Sulfuric Acid (H_2SO_4)

In its pure state, sulfuric acid is an oily, colorless, and odorless liquid with a strongly acidic taste.

Its affinity for water is such that it carbonizes organic substances, leading to the formation of this compound at the expense of the oxygen and hydrogen contained in such substances. The ease with which this acid, better known as "oil of vitriol," can be obtained, and its common use in arts and industries, explains the relative frequency of accidental and intentional poisonings for suicidal purposes.

Symptoms of poisoning. - As soon as the poison is ingested, symptoms arise with formidable rapidity. The patient reports a burning, excruciating pain from the mouth to the stomach, a pain that elicits cries and throws them into the most frightening anguish.

Vomiting is frequent, consisting of brownish, mucous, and bloody matter, so acidic that it fizzes when hitting the floor. These generally occur immediately after ingestion; in some cases, they are delayed by half an hour or more, and in others, they are entirely absent due to the paralyzing action of the poison. There is also continuous, intense pain in the epigastrium; the eyes are sunken; the lips and mouth contours are covered with gray or brown spots or scabs; consciousness remains unaltered. Body temperature is lowered; the pulse is small, hard, rare, or frequent; breathing is difficult; swallowing is painful; excessive salivation and a severe sense of suffocation are also observed. The abdomen is mostly swollen and tender to the touch; there are no bowel movements; diarrhea rarely occurs, with black stools due to blood; urine is suppressed. Agitation becomes extreme; strength diminishes rapidly; death occurs within a few hours, at most in three or four days, due to collapse or edema of the glottis, rarely due to acute peritonitis from perforation.

Sometimes the corrosive poison enters the respiratory tract; in these cases, death by suffocation is the prompt consequence.

The *course* of sulfuric acid poisoning is not always so acute; in some cases, either due to the smaller dose of poison ingested or its lower concentration, only a more or less intense gastroenteritis can be noticed. These mild cases may end in slow recovery, after a gradual detachment of necrotized parts, but patients often die of wasting in a few weeks or months.

Anatomical lesions. - In fatal cases, post-mortem examination shows, in addition to black scabs on the lips and inside the mouth, more or less extensive and deep brown streaks along the length of the esophagus. The gastric mucosa is usually black, or shows here and there red or black patches that can be peeled off in strips. Other times the entire wall appears carbonized in all its thickness, or completely perforated in one or more points. In this case, the acid has penetrated the abdominal cavity, exerting its corrosive action on various organs: liver, spleen, mesentery, and even the aorta. The intestine is generally healthy, at most it may show some traces of inflammation. The kidneys show signs of intense parenchymal inflammation; the bladder is empty or contains only a small amount of bloody urine. The heart contains numerous clots; black coagulated blood was found by *Grisolle* in the iliac veins, by *Tardieu* in the femoral arteries, in the vessels of the stomach and mesentery. If the poisoning did not end in death in the initial period, extensive scarring formations of the parts directly attacked by the corrosive liquid are observed.

When the course of intoxication was relatively slow, the stomach may show no other lesion than that of chronic inflammation, characterized by a mamillated appearance of the mucosa and a narrowing of the organ. *Tardieu* saw the stomach of an adult reduced to the volume of that of a child; the narrowing can reach such a point that an egg can fill the cavity of the ventricle. Other times, a true atrophy of the entire digestive tube was noted.

Nitric Acid (HNO_3)

Nitric acid, also known as *azotic* acid, is a colorless, extremely corrosive liquid that turns yellow when exposed to light. Like sulfuric acid, it is widely used in various industries. It is especially used by hat makers, porcelain painters, and, when combined with hydrochloric acid, by metal engravers.

Chemists, laboratory assistants, and workers in chemical manufacturing or in the production of fulminating cotton are highly exposed to the harmful effects that nitric acid fumes can cause. *Taylor* cites many cases where the inhalation of these fumes led to shortness of breath, violent coughing, and rapidly fatal suffocation.

Upon autopsy, lung congestion, blood acidity, and inflammation of the endocardium and the inner lining of the large vessels were found.

Symptoms and Course of Poisoning. - The symptoms closely resemble those of sulfuric acid poisoning. Characteristic ochre-yellow spots may be found on the lips; the inside of the mouth and throat appear opaque white, due to thickened and severely cauterized mucosa; the surface of the tongue is very white, showing yellowish spots; the teeth may sometimes be shaky, with yellow crowns. Yellowish spots can also appear on the chin or fingers. The tonsils are swollen. Severe pain, initially localized in the upper abdomen, rapidly spreads to nearby areas, accompanied by vomiting of highly acidic, viscous, sometimes bloody substances. The abdomen becomes distended and painful; bloody diarrhea may appear soon after, although sometimes there is obstinate constipation. The voice becomes hoarse; a violent cough with bloody sputum may occur if the acid penetrates the larynx. Other symptoms include shortness of breath, painful urination, irregular and frequent weak pulse, extreme fatigue, and lowered body temperature. Cognitive function eventually becomes impaired, and delirium precedes death, which can occur after one or several days, or even less than two hours if the acid penetrates the airways. However, the course is not always so acute, nor the outcome always fatal.

Anatomical Lesions. - The epithelium of the oral, lingual, and esophageal mucosa is lifted, wrinkled, and gray-violet, sometimes replaced by a crust of a rancid color. The stomach contents are dense, viscous, and bloody; the mucosa is red, softened, and scattered with dark spots formed by submucous ecchymosis. In very rare cases, the stomach was found to be perforated. Ulcerations may also occur in the small intestine, and sometimes gastroenteric inflammation was seen to spread to the peritoneum. Frequently, the laryngeal mucosa is found to be red, swollen, devoid of its epithelium, and edematous; the trachea is inflamed, and the lungs congested. The heart mostly contains fluid and black blood. In cases that had a slower course, only the characteristic signs of chronic gastritis with mucosal hypertrophy and pyloric stenosis, or more or less extensive esophageal stenosis, can be found.

Hydrochloric Acid (HCl)

This concentrated acid is a colorless liquid, with a very penetrating odor and an extremely acidic taste, emitting dense vapors when exposed to air. It is widely used in chemical analysis, for preserving timber, for softening ivory; it is also frequently used in the manufacturing of gelatins, carbonated water, and in a multitude of other industries.

Like the preceding acids, it is a very potent poison.

Symptoms of Poisoning. - The symptoms are identical to

those produced by nitric acid, differing only in the special grayish hue of the stains found around the mouth, on the lips, and inside the oral cavity, and by the formation of dense pseudomembranes on the mucous membranes attacked by the acid.

Anatomical Lesions. - Upon autopsy, *Taylor* found the oral and pharyngeal mucosa to be white, softened, and corroded here and there by the corrosive liquid; the esophagus mucosa was red, inflamed, while that of the stomach was destroyed near the pylorus and black, escharotic in the rest of its extension. *Tardieu* reports an interesting case of a 15-day-old baby, whose mother, trying to cure him of thrush, cauterized the inside of his mouth with fuming hydrochloric acid. As expected, the sucking movements caused the baby to swallow a small amount of the acid, which was sufficient to kill him. On autopsy, the esophageal mucosa was found destroyed, and the channel was lined with a grayish pseudomembrane.

Prognosis of Poisonings by Concentrated Acids - It is serious in most cases; the saying by *Zacchia* applies to such poisonings: «*Venena, nisi occidant, relinquunt semper aliquam noxam et morbos diuturnos*» ("Venom, unless it kills, always leaves behind some harm and long-term diseases"), because even if a fatal outcome is averted, there is little hope for the future. Scar tissue, contracting over time, causes severe stenosis, especially of the esophagus, which often makes feeding the patient inevitable through a gastric fistula.

Treatment. - It is prudent not to resort to a gastric tube, to avoid the danger of producing lacerations in already altered tissues; emetics are also absolutely to be avoided. Alkaline carbonates should not be used to neutralize the acids, as the carbonic acid produced by them could excessively expand the gastric walls and cause rupture. Burnt magnesia (several spoonfuls in water) is the most frequently used antidote; it saturates the acids well, forming salts that are harmless or at most mildly purgative. If this metallic oxide is not available, common soda soap can be used. For sulfuric acid poisoning, *Bamberger* prefers lime water to magnesia itself, prescribing several spoonfuls every five minutes. Later, symptomatic treatment will be given, administering small pieces of ice, mucilaginous drinks to reduce gastrointestinal irritation; antiseptic gargles and mouthwashes, etc. The diet will be light (milk, eggs, etc.); irritating foods and alcoholic beverages will be avoided. Esophageal stenosis will be methodically treated with probes.

For accidents caused by nitrous vapors and sulfuric acid, skin revulsives (mustard plasters on the chest, etc.), narcotics, expectorants, and oxygen inhalations will be used.

II. Concentrated Vegetable Acids

Oxalic Acid ($C^2H^2O^4$)

This acid crystallizes in colorless prisms and is highly soluble in water and alcohol. It is rarely found in a free state but seems to occur in the "Boletus sulfureus." It resembles certain medical salts, such as magnesium sulfate, and can easily be a cause of accidental poisoning. It is used by dyers, textile printers, and straw hat manufacturers; many households use it daily for cleaning copper cookware. A dose of just 2 grams proved fatal for a 16-year-old boy.

A noteworthy feature is that this acid is more active when diluted.

Symptoms of poisoning. - Immediately after ingestion, the first symptom is a burning pain in the stomach and sometimes also in the throat, often followed by vomiting of dark, sometimes bloody, matter. In a case reported by *Deane*, the vomit consisted of pure, vermilion blood. The abdomen is tense and painful; the pulse is small, irregular, almost imperceptible. The body is covered in cold, sticky sweat; the patient feels numbness and tingling in the limbs; in other cases, there is a complete loss of consciousness, tonic and clonic convulsions. Sugar may be found in the urine; often there is anuria, due to the blockage of the urine ducts by the accumulation of calcium oxalate crystals. Death, due to heart or nerve center paralysis, can occur within a few minutes (*Orfila*), a few hours; more rarely within a few days.

Anatomical lesions. - The mucosa from the mouth to the stomach generally appears white; the gastric contents are brown, often acidic and gelatinous; the soft mucosa of this organ appears sometimes inflamed and eroded, or even gangrenous and destroyed. The blood is vermilion, as are the tissues supplied by a rich capillary network. *Welck* observed pulmonary congestion, with engorgement of the heart and large vessels.

Treatment. - *Husemann* recommends calcium saccharate in these cases. Lime water, powdered eggshells, which combine with the acid to form insoluble calcium oxalate, will also be useful.

Magnesia will also be helpful; symptomatic treatment should naturally not be neglected.

(APPENDIX)

Potassium Bisoxalate
(Wood Sorrel Salt. $K^2G^2O^4$)

This salt exists in the juice of various Rumex plants, and especially in that of Oxalis acetosella; it is used to clean metals and to remove rust and ink stains.

Accidental poisonings have been caused by its resemblance to cream of tartar. Its toxicity is greater than that of saltpeter; a dose of 12-16 grams can be fatal for an adult.

Symptoms of poisoning. - These are very similar to those of oxalic acid poisoning, with death occurring within a few hours. However, there are instances of recovery, such as the case cited by Taylor of a twenty-year-old woman who had ingested a 30-gram dose, with extremely violent symptoms.

Anatomical Lesions. - At autopsy, considerable congestion of the lungs was found, hemorrhages in various organs, and a very bright vermilion color of the tissues and blood. The stomach may, in some cases, show no signs of inflammation (*Tardieu*).

Treatmen. - Lime water (100-200 grams), light magnesia; symptomatic treatment.

Acetic Acid ($C^2H^4O^2$)

It is a colorless, clear liquid with a strong vinegar odor and a very pungent taste. It dissolves protein substances as well as epithelial cells and the epidermis, producing almost liquid, oily scabs.

When ingested, it leads to the phenomena of severe gastroenteritis, with excoriation of the mucosa, intense fever, collapse, and death. At autopsy, in addition to the inflammation of the gastrointestinal tract, a lacquer-like coloration of the blood is noted, due to the destruction of hemoglobin and the transfer of hematin into the serum (*Mitscherlich*).

Wine vinegar, which is a more or less diluted solution of acetic acid, acts similarly but with much less potency.

Treatment. - Light magnesia, lime water, mucilaginous drinks; symptomatic treatment.

Citric Acid ($C^6H^8O^7$) and Tartaric Acid ($C^4H^6O^6$)

Citric acid crystallizes in rhomboidal prisms, is soluble in water and alcohol, odorless, and has a very acidic taste. It combines with nitric acid to form oxalic acid.

It is widely distributed in nature; it is found in a free state, either alone or associated with tartaric and malic acids, in most acidic fruits, especially in oranges, lemons, and citrons. It is widely used, besides in medicine, in dyeing to isolate safflower red and to brighten the tones of this coloring substance; to prepare a tin solution that gives beautiful scarlets with cochineal; bookbinders use it to prepare an iron solution that gives leather a marbled appearance; chemists use it to test for phosphates. Chronic poisoning cases occur, characterized by skin coloration and abnormal production of corneal cells, in addition to bronchitis, stomach problems, weight loss, and anemia.

Tartaric acid is a white, solid substance, crystallized in hexagonal prisms terminated by triangular pyramids, soluble in alcohol and more so in water, sparingly in ether.

It is widely used in medicine, chemical analysis, dyeing, and textile printing.

Intoxication from these two acids produces the same symptoms as that caused by acetic acid; the treatment is identical.

III. Caustic Alkalis

Caustic Potash (*Potassium Hydroxide*, KHO)

Commercial potash or potassium hydroxide is a white substance, greasy to the touch, with a urinous and caustic taste, extremely soluble in water.

Its use is very popular and frequent; it suffices to mention its consumption by laundresses and soap factories. However, poisoning cases are extremely rare; its immediate action in the mouth makes malicious or accidental poisoning very difficult, and suicides generally resort to other toxins. 10 or 20 grams of this substance can cause fatal incidents in an adult.

Symptoms of Poisoning. - Ingestion of the poison is immediately followed by a burning sensation, a pungent and urinous taste in the mouth, warmth, and tightness in the throat, along the esophagus, and in the stomach.

This intense pain is accompanied by nausea and vomiting of highly alkaline substances, often mixed with blood. Profuse, bloody diarrhea soon occurs, along with excruciating colic, agonizing epigastric pain, extreme anxiety, convulsive tremors, or actual limb convulsions.

Often, these symptoms are joined by those of acute peritonitis due to stomach perforation. Vomiting and diarrhea cease, the temperature drops, the pulse becomes increasingly rare, bloating is extreme, consciousness is altered, and death can occur within a few hours, with or without nervous symptoms. When, as more frequently happens, the outcome is not so rapid, patients generally succumb after three or four months due to severe wasting, a consequence of chronic inflammation of the digestive organs.

Anatomical Lesions. - The post-mortem examination reveals less profound but more extensive alterations than those caused by corrosive acids in the mucosa of the mouth, pharynx, and esophagus, which were found to be softened, detached, and inflamed in the form of dark chocolate-colored spots, sometimes almost black. The same alterations can be found on the mucosa of the larynx and trachea. In the stomach, a sort of wet, colliquative gangrene is noted, affecting the entire organ and all its layers, which are sometimes perforated. In cases where the course was more chronic, Tardieu observed ulcerative or suppurative inflammation of the mucosa, esophageal stenosis, with a waxy appearance of its walls, and above the constricted point, a sort of diverticulum where food was lodged.

Treatment. - Large amounts of acidulated water to neutralize all the free alkali and induce vomiting; albuminous water, milk, abundant mucilaginous drinks. Treatment of various symptoms.

Caustic Soda (*Sodium Hydroxide*, NaOH)

The solution of sodium hydroxide, or caustic soda, commonly used by laundresses, in soap factories, glassworks, etc., has very strong caustic properties. Its corrosive effects are similar to those produced by potash. Materials expelled with vomit, saliva, and intestinal content have a smell of lye and are strongly alkaline; urine can have the same reaction. The treatment is the same as for potash poisoning.

Liquid Ammonia (*Volatile Alkali*)

This is obtained by dissolving ammonia gas (NH_3) in water.

It is a colorless, clear liquid with an extremely penetrating, distinctive, and caustic taste. Ammonia is widely used in industries, serving in the production of imitation pearls, in dyeing to dissolve carmine and increase the solubility of some coloring substances, in baking to make dough lighter and softer, and in tobacco manufacturing to enhance aroma. It is toxic even in moderate doses; 30 grams are enough to kill an adult.

Symptoms of Poisoning. - Ingestion of the caustic is immediately followed by a sense of throat constriction, agonizing stomach pain, and soon after, excessive salivation, repeated viscous vomiting streaked with blood, strongly alkaline; intense colic pain accompanied by diarrheal discharges, scanty and bloody urine. The face expresses extreme anguish, the voice is hoarse, eyes are fierce and bloodshot, and lips are significantly swollen. In cases where the liquid has penetrated the nasal passages and larynx, there are episodes of suffocation, abundant and loud bronchial rattling, and severe shortness of breath. Death can occur within a few hours or days; however, even violent symptoms can subside, and complete recovery can occur in a short time.

Anatomical Lesions. - Autopsy shows intense inflammation of the mucosa of the upper digestive tract, which may also present dry and yellowish scabs. In the intestine, traces of inflammation can sometimes be found, with more or less superficial ulcers or submucosal hemorrhages. The liver is softened, yellowish, and greasy when cut, with bruising under the capsule. The kidneys may also show fatty degeneration. Pseudomembranous croup has often been observed on the bronchial mucosa, while the lungs appeared congested or even inflamed. The blood is fluid, uncoagulable.

Inhaling ammonia gas leads to violent reflex phenomena:

sneezing, coughing, inspiratory cramps, episodes of suffocation, and nervous disturbances (dizziness, etc.).

Treatment. - In recent cases, a gastric pump can be advantageously used. Acidulated (citric or acetic acid) and mucilaginous drinks, milk, anti-inflammatory agents, fatty emulsions, and narcotics are all beneficial.

In cases of suffocation due to ammonia gas, the patient should be moved to fresh air, and bronchial irritation will be alleviated with steam inhalations.

IV - Silver Nitrate (AgNO^3)

Poisoning from silver salts is extremely rare due to their very low absorption by the body.

Silver nitrate poisoning most commonly occurs accidentally through the ingestion of a piece of caustic material (also known as "lunar caustic") used for cauterizing the throat; in other cases, it happens through ingestion of this salt in concentrated solution.

In these instances, violent stomach irritation is observed, along with intense pain, vomiting, and diarrhea. In the most severe cases, symptoms of acute peritonitis due to perforation may manifest. The vomited material initially appears whitish in color but quickly turns brown, and then black.

Treatment. - The antidotes are heavily salted water, milk, and albumin.

IRRITANT POISONS

I - Mineral Irritant Poisons

Iodine (I)

This metalloid, extracted from seaweed, is solid with a metallic luster: it appears in the form of grayish flakes or large, very dark violet octahedral crystals. It has a distinctive smell, similar to that of chlorine, but much less penetrating, and a bitter taste. Barely soluble in water, it dissolves easily in alcohol, ether, gasoline, chloroform, and essential oils.

Upon heating, it releases vapors of a beautiful violet color. It is widely used in medicine, especially in alcoholic solution form. Iodine initially irritates and then paralyzes respiration, it paralyzes the nervous centers, and depletes the normal alkali of the tissues, causing the poisoning to resemble that caused by acids (*Pellacani*).

Acute Poisoning (*Acute Iodism*). - This occurs following the ingestion of toxic doses of pure iodine or its tincture, of iodine compounds (potassium iodide); it has also been observed as a consequence of injections of significant amounts of iodine tincture into natural cavities, ovarian cysts, etc.

Symptoms of poisoning. - Immediately after ingestion,

symptoms due to irritation of the digestive mucosa appear: an acrid and burning taste in the mouth and a sense of scalding in the throat with intense thirst, vomiting of brownish-yellow material, in which blue spots can be seen due to the presence of starchy substances (bread, etc.); a sense of warmth in the stomach, intense colic pains. Subsequently, more severe symptoms develop: pallor and coldness of the skin, cyanosis of the lips, cheeks, and extremities; a small and frequent pulse, oliguria with albuminous urine, sometimes hemoglobinuria; the temperature remains normal or is slightly elevated. After 3 or 4 days, if these symptoms have not faded, the appearance of cutaneous rashes (roseola, pustules, urticaria, erythema, eczema, erysipelas) is noted. Usually, there are also symptoms from the respiratory system: rhinitis, dyspnea, cough with catarrhal or even bloody sputum. In some cases, metrorrhagia was observed. Chemical analysis reveals iodine in the urine, saliva, milk, and nasal mucus as soon as 5 minutes after ingestion.

Nervous disturbances of varying intensity are not uncommon: headache, ringing in the ears, dizziness, fainting, insomnia, great agitation, convulsions. After a week or more, there is a progressive improvement of all symptoms, with slow healing; but it may also happen that death occurs quite suddenly during convalescence.

Anatomical lesions. - In addition to more or less severe inflammation of the mucous membranes, the blood's coloring matter is found to be dissolved; urine and pleural exudates appear red.

Treatment. - Administer plentiful starch decoction,

albuminous water, mucilaginous drinks, milk, and starch enemas; induce vomiting with the ingestion of hot water or with hypodermic injection of apomorphine. Later, recourse will be taken to sedatives and anti-inflammatory treatments.

Iodine vapors, when they come into contact with the mucous membranes, cause irritation and inflammation; tearing, sneezing, acrid and warm taste in the mouth, prickling and soreness in the throat, coughing can be noticed. Bronchitis can be a consequence; bronchorrhagia is not rare in predisposed individuals. Fresh air and steam inhalations are the main therapeutic indications.

Iodoform (CHI^3) is a substance with a beautiful sulfur yellow color, with a strong and characteristic odor, insoluble in water, but soluble in alcohol, ether, chloroform, gasoline, glycerin, and both fixed and volatile oils.

Poisoning is usually caused by dressings with iodoform on wounds, sores, burns. *Elicher* observed intoxication following an oophorectomy in which only 6 grams of iodoform had been dusted on the stump.

Symptoms of poisoning. - They can be divided into general and local. The former include anorexia, coated tongue, the taste of iodoform in the mouth. Subsequent nervous disturbances appear: restlessness, insomnia, delirium. The pulse is small and frequent. In more severe cases, there is great excitement, hallucinations, delirium, very frequent pulse, subfebrile state or high fever, loss of consciousness, death in severe collapse. The duration of these symptoms can vary from one day to over a month.

The local symptoms consist of eczema or erythema.

Anatomical lesions. - Autopsy shows fatty degeneration of the heart, liver, kidneys, edema of the pia mater or chronic leptomeningitis. Iodoform is a protoplasmic poison; it paralyzes the movement of white blood cells and prevents their diapedesis, thus opposing suppuration.

Treatment. - Immediately remove the dressing and any iodoform that may be on the wound. Administer alkaline substances (5-10% aqueous solution of potassium bicarbonate); for the rest, symptomatic treatment.

Ingestion of iodoform in nature or suspended in water only produces slow and mild effects; on the contrary, if swallowed in solution, it produces rapid and dangerous effects even in relatively weak doses. *Oberlander* has cited numerous cases of poisoning due to the administration, for eighty consecutive days, of a pill containing 50 centigrams of iodoform; the ingestion of 5 grams of iodoform, taken in a week, caused symptoms of intoxication. The elderly and those with heart disease feel the effects of the drug more than others.

Symptoms. - Usually consist of nausea, vomiting and diarrhea, shallow breathing, increased temperature, drowsiness or manic excitement. In a later period, the symptoms of collapse appear (decrease in cardiac activity and temperature, etc.); death can occur due to cardiac or respiratory paralysis.

Anatomical lesions. - Fatty degeneration of the heart, kidneys, liver, etc.; congestion of the lungs.

Treatment. - Gastric lavage in recent cases; treatment of the various symptoms.

Chronic Iodism. - Chronic iodine poisoning is usually observed after excessively prolonged use of iodine or iodides. At first, symptoms of irritation of the mucous membranes of the digestive and respiratory tracts appear: nausea, loss of appetite, ptyalism, retching, digestive disturbances, colic pains with diarrhea, rhinitis, angina, bronchitis, bronchopneumonia, pleuritis.

Conjunctivitis is also often observed; the appearance of skin rashes (acne, erythema) is very frequent. From the nervous system, there is restlessness, general overexcitation, heart palpitations, limb tremors. After a certain time, the patients complain of great weakness, become cachectic, and the skin takes on a characteristic yellow-earthy color.

Treatment. - The first indication is to suspend the iodine medications. Internally, sodium bicarbonate and sodium sulfide should be prescribed. Hot sulfur baths will be very beneficial. The diet should be strengthening, predominantly meat-based. *Ehrlich* asserts that the internal use of sulfanilic acid often rapidly dispels the symptoms of intoxication; *Briquet* recommends belladonna against stubborn nasopharyngeal incidents.

Bromine (Br.).

Bromine is a liquid at room temperature, with a reddish-brown color; at 58°C, it emits yellowish vapors. It has an extremely irritating and unpleasant odor, and a very caustic taste. This element is slightly soluble in water; soluble in alcohol and especially in ether.

Inhalation of bromine vapors produces the same symptoms as those caused by chlorine vapors.

When *ingested,* it is highly toxic; indeed, just one drop diluted in 15 grams of water can cause salivation, diarrhea, headache, and general weakness. Larger doses result in symptoms of violent inflammation and cauterization of the gastro-enteric mucosa, mydriasis, stupor and coma, convulsions, death due to cardiac paralysis.

Treatment. - Alkaline solutions (potassium or sodium carbonate); symptomatic treatment.

Prolonged use of bromides (especially potassium or sodium bromide) often leads to chronic intoxication (*chronic bromism*), a type of cachexia characterized by severe muscular weakness, intellectual inertia, forgetfulness, reduced reflex movements, anorexia, diarrhea, sexual weakness or impotence, and the appearance of a skin rash (bromic acne).

In the most severe cases, there is noted aphonia, muscular paralysis, abolition of reflexes, deafness, blindness, loss of taste, hallucinations of sight and hearing, cretinism or idiocy, lowering of temperature, progressive weakness, and ultimately cessation of cardiac contractions. Atonic ulcers appear on the legs.

Treatment. - Immediately discontinue the use of the drug, facilitate its elimination from the body (diuretics, diaphoretics, warm beverages). Support the patient's strength. Treatment of the various symptoms.

Chlorine (Cl.).

This metalloid is gaseous at room temperature, with a yellow-green color, highly soluble in water, and has a suffocating odor. It acts as a strong oxidizing agent; by reacting with organic substances, it profoundly modifies them due to its affinity for the hydrogen they contain. It is often used in industries to bleach linen or cotton fabrics and in medicine as a disinfectant.

Inhalation of chlorine gas exerts a violent action on the mucous membranes of the respiratory tract. *Symptoms* include tearing, sneezing, a sense of constriction and suffocation, dyspnea, and convulsive cough with sero-sanguineous expectoration, transient spasm of the glottis, sensorial dullness, and drowsiness. If exposure to chlorine is prolonged, bronchitis, croupous tracheitis, and bronchopneumonia can develop. *Treatment* involves moving the patient to the open air and having them inhale water vapor or ammonia. Chloroform and narcotics may also be useful.

Workers routinely exposed to chlorine inhalations show symptoms of anemia, weight loss; chronic stomatitis and pharyngitis, and dyspepsia.

Chlorine water ingested into the stomach causes severe irritation that can progress to corrosion of the digestive tract mucosa. In such cases, albuminous water, mucilaginous beverages, and plenty of milk, etc., should be administered.

Phosphorus (Ph.).

Phosphorus, which is extracted from the ash of bones where it exists as calcium neutral phosphate, is a metalloid that is solid at room temperature, soft enough to retain a fingernail impression, insoluble in water, and only slightly soluble in alcohol and ether; however, it dissolves very well in oils and other fatty substances. It is yellowish and transparent, luminous in the dark due to slow combustion, and possesses an exceedingly potent toxic power. When heated for a few hours in an inert gas at temperatures of 235-250 degrees Celsius, it undergoes a significant change: it turns red, becomes opaque, and is no longer poisonous.

Acute poisoning. - This can occur through ingestion of raw phosphorus, phosphoric paste used for exterminating vermin, or a solution of match heads (ten matchsticks can be lethal). In some cases, it may result from the misuse of aphrodisiac medicines, with phosphorus as the main ingredient. Generally, such poisonings are self-inflicted; criminal and accidental poisonings are made much more difficult by the garlic-like odor and the nauseating, extremely disgusting taste of this substance.

The lethal dose is highly variable. *Kessler* observed the death of a seven-week-old child within 3-4 hours after ingesting 20 milligrams of phosphorus. A 52-year-old woman consumed 60 milligrams of phosphorus over four days and died three days after the last dose of 30 milligrams. *Falck* and *Husemann* consider a dose of 0.03-0.18 grams to be lethal or very dangerous.

The rapidity and severity of symptoms are greatly influenced by the form in which the poison is ingested or administered; 5 centigrams of phosphorus in solution can be a lethal dose, while 10-20 centigrams may be required if the substance is in fine powder. Large fragments can pass through the entire digestive tract almost unchanged.

Symptoms of Poisoning. - The first to appear are those of acute gastro-enteric catarrh: nausea, burps smelling of phosphorus, vomit that is luminous in the dark and sometimes mixed with blood, colicky pains, constipation, or diarrhea with phosphorescent and sometimes bloody evacuations. These symptoms, of varying duration, can offer a remission for 2-3 days, after which the signs of absorption appear: increased heart rate and respiration, fever, restlessness, prostration, insomnia, pain or tingling at the extremities, anesthesia, paralysis, lethargy, convulsions, death within a few days, rarely in a few hours or after a week. Urinalysis shows an increase in urea in the urine and the presence of albumin, hemoglobin, cylinders, and sometimes leucine and tyrosine.

In children, death may occur within 4-6 hours, with no other symptoms than some vomiting followed by drowsiness and convulsions.

Anatomical Lesions. - In addition to signs of inflammation, the digestive mucosa may show ecchymotic plaques; tiny ulcerations appear in the stomach and intestines.

The stomach contents have a bloody coloration, the mucosa is swollen, and the epithelial cells of the gastric glands are in fatty degeneration (*Virchow*'s glandular gastritis). The liver is enlarged, with a whitish-yellow or intense yellow color; the yellowish areas are often mixed with red-brown ones, giving the organ a marbled appearance.

There is also fatty degeneration of the kidneys, spleen, myocardium, uterus, trunk muscles, and vascular walls. The lungs, intestine, kidneys, uterus, and serous membranes are usually the sites of more or less considerable hemorrhages. The blood is altered, black, and oily.

The external appearance of the corpse presents nothing particular, only sometimes subcutaneous ecchymoses are found.

Treatment. - In recent cases, when the poison has not yet been absorbed, gastric lavage will be performed, and emetics administered. As antidotes, unrectified turpentine oil (30-40 drops in a mucilaginous potion) is prescribed. According to *Personne*, phosphorus becomes toxic because, by absorbing oxygen, it prevents the oxygenation of the blood, and turpentine essence would be a true antidote, as it prevents this oxygen absorption by the phosphorus. Solutions of copper sulfate are also recommended; better yet is diluted potassium permanganate (0.5-1:100). Fatty substances, which dissolve phosphorus and facilitate its absorption, must be absolutely avoided.

Chronic Poisoning. - Workers in match factories, who inhale phosphorus vapors daily, are subject to a special cachexia known as chronic phosphorism. The severity of intoxication varies according to age, constitution, individual predisposition, etc.

Symptoms. - Chronic phosphorism presents common symptoms: ptyalism, garlic-like breath odor, albuminuria, anemia, muscular and cardiac weakness, severe prostration, forgetfulness, neurasthenia, subicteric tint of the skin. Urine and saliva contain phosphorus.

The special symptoms, depending on individual predisposition, usually include: nephritis, interstitial hepatitis, chronic enteric catarrh with stubborn diarrhea, odontalgia, fragility of bones, periostitis, necrosis of the lower jaw, more rarely of the upper jaws. These necroses usually start at a decayed tooth.

Treatment. - The patient must at least temporarily leave the manufacturing environment and go to stay in the countryside or mountains to lead an active life. A nutritious diet, milk treatment, turpentine-based preparations, and hydrotherapy will also be very useful.

Prophylaxis would mainly consist of good ventilation in factories and legal prohibition of the use of white phosphorus.

Arsenic (As.).

This metal is solid at ordinary temperatures, brittle, with a steel-gray color and very bright luster. It is insoluble in water, odorless, and tasteless; when heated it volatilizes without melting, and when thrown on burning coals it gives off a strong garlic-like smell.

There are many arsenical compounds used in the arts and industries. It suffices to mention Schweinfurt green (copper acetoarsenite) and Scheele's green (copper arsenite) used in dyeing wallpapers, fabrics, and artificial flowers; orpiment (arsenic trisulfide $As_2 S_3$), and realgar (red sulfide $As_2 S_2$) which, besides being used in painting, are also used in the preparation of many hair removal pastes and powders; among the pharmaceutical preparations are Fowler's solution (potassium arsenite solution), Pearson's solution (sodium arsenate solution), various caustic pastes, and white arsenic (arsenic trioxide $As_2 O_3$) or arsenious acid. In commerce, there is a known substance, "poudre aux mouches," which contains arsenic and arsenious acid. All these compounds possess a very strong toxic power; 1-3 centigrams of arsenious acid can cause symptoms of poisoning, 15-20 centigrams are enough to cause death.

Evidently, arsenical compounds, with such widespread, varied, and frequent use, often lead to professional or accidental poisonings, or even criminal ones due to the ease of procuring these poisons and their almost non-existent taste.

Waters from manufacturing, workshops, and laboratories that use arsenicals, when carelessly discharged, have often poisoned well waters. Candles dyed with arsenical green, or with wicks containing arsenious acid, release arsenical vapors when burned. *Ritter* reports a case where vapors from a white Bengal fire (also called Indian fire), prepared with orpiment and lit in a high and narrow courtyard, produced poisoning symptoms in the tenants of the third floor. In Troppau (Bohemia), many people recently fell ill with poisoning symptoms after drinking soda water (Sodawasser) from a factory that had used highly arsenical sulfuric acid to prepare this water.

Acute Poisoning. - This usually occurs through the *application on the skin* or ingestion of soluble arsenical substances.

With the skin application of a concentrated arsenical compound, after 10-12 hours, acute pain and erythema at the application site and symptoms of absorption arise: vomiting and diarrhea, fever, epistaxis, and more or less intense nervous disturbances; in the most severe cases, collapse and death within a few days. *Leprince* observed the case of a young girl with a breast tumor who turned to the treatments of a quack; this person gave her a "pomade" and an "aqua." Five days after using these remedies, the young girl died and medical expertise established that the pomade contained orpiment, and the aqua contained arsenious acid.

According to *Sklarck*, arsenic decreases the excitability of the nerve centers in the spinal cord; it first stimulates and then paralyzes the respiratory center in the medulla oblongata.

In *acute poisoning by ingestion,* symptoms of a violent, cholera-like gastroenteritis emerge within an hour, and sometimes even earlier. These include a sensation of heat and constriction in the throat, repeated vomiting initially smelling of rotten eggs or garlic, intense colicky pain, rice–water–like diarrheal discharges, headache, dizziness, facial cyanosis; collapse, general paralysis; blood and albumin are sometimes found in the urine. Other times, the only symptoms may be mild fainting followed by drowsiness; death occurs within 12–20 hours, due to cardiac or respiratory paralysis.

However, in most cases the course is not so rapid; after 1–2 days, the vomiting ceases and there appears to be an improvement in all symptoms, with only dyspnea, pulse irregularities, and difficulty swallowing persisting, along with severe weakness. Fever often sets in with restlessness and insomnia, and between the 2nd and 5th day of illness, cutaneous eruptions (petechiae, pustules, urticaria, erysipelas on the face or genitals) may appear, hair and nails may fall out, and jaundice is rarely seen. This improvement is usually temporary; the pulse becomes increasingly weak and frequent, delirium, coma, and death ensue within a few days. In some cases, however, good care and especially individual resistance can avert this fatal outcome; recovery occurs slowly over two weeks or even two or three months.

Anatomical lesions. - The gastroenteric mucosa generally shows, in addition to signs of inflammation, erosions, ulcerations, hemorrhages, swelling of solitary follicles. The lungs are simply congested or the site of extensive subpleural ecchymoses; ecchymoses are also typically found beneath the pericardium or the endocardium. The liver, kidneys, heart, and muscles often show fatty degeneration.

Arsenic can be traced in all organs; it is also found in the placenta and in the fetus.

Treatment. - The use of the stomach pump, combined with the administration of emetics, will be very useful in recent cases. The antidote is *hydrated iron oxide* (2-4 tablespoons every half hour in warm water).

Known as "antidotum arsenici", a mixture of 60 parts liquid ferric sulfate in 420 of water, and 7 parts of burnt magnesia in 120 of water is prepared at the moment of use. This mixture forms hydrated iron oxide, which in the presence of arsenic results in the formation of insoluble arsenite of iron.

The administration of burnt magnesia and egg-white water (6-8 egg whites in a liter of water) is also very beneficial.

Chronic Poisoning. - Chronic arsenical poisoning may be observed after excessively prolonged treatment with arsenic preparations, or as a chronic form of an acute poisoning; more often, it occurs among workers in arsenic mines, glass factories, textile factories (where more than 8 grams of arsenious acid were found in one meter of fabric), artificial flower makers, producers of colored papers, and taxidermists.

Symptoms. - They generally begin with conjunctivitis, a sense of constriction and dryness in the throat, and slight hoarseness. This is followed by chronic gastroenteritis, with nervous disorders: headache, insomnia, neuralgia, tremors, and paralysis of the limbs. Alopecia, the earthy pallor of the skin, eczema, and cutaneous ulcerations, hectic fever, and marasmus complete the nosological picture of this serious cachexia.

Treatment. - Promptly remove the patient from the sources of poisoning and treat the various morbid manifestations.

«*Arsenic Eaters*». According to *Tschudi*, the habit of consuming arsenic is quite common in some regions of Lower Austria and Styria, especially in the mountains bordering Hungary. They purchase it under the name "*hedri*" from herbalists and itinerant merchants, who in turn acquire it from Hungarian glassworks laborers, or from veterinarians, charlatans, etc. Their aim is twofold: to become more agile, better suited to endure the harsh mountain life, and at the same time to acquire a healthy, flourishing appearance, which they often achieve in a surprising manner.

However, the number of deaths from poisoning is not insignificant, although it is very difficult to compile statistics, because the arsenic eater generally does not reveal his habit to anyone, partly out of shame, partly for fear of the penalties that the law imposes on illegitimate possessors of this poison.

They start with a very small dose (less than half a grain) and for a long time do not exceed it, taking it in the morning on an empty stomach several times a week. When they have become sufficiently accustomed, they gradually increase the dose, thus coming to ingest relatively enormous quantities with impunity. It is noteworthy that if the use of arsenic is interrupted, either due to a lack of the toxin or for any other reason, symptoms similar to those of mild arsenical intoxication always appear. There is only one effective way to counter all these phenomena: the immediate return to the use of arsenic.

Lead (Pb.).

Taking into account not only deliberate or criminal poisonings (which are quite rare in truth), but also, and above all, accidental and occupational poisonings, we can assert that intoxications by lead or its compounds are far more frequent and numerous than those that could be caused by any other poisonous substance.

Food preserves (meat, legumes, anchovies, various sauces) enclosed in iron cans that contain lead, or soldered with tin that contains this metal, candied fruits, chocolate, and confections wrapped in so-called "tin foil" can become impregnated with lead; cases of poisoning caused by tea wrapped in lead foil were observed in 1886 in Odessa. *Flinger* analyzed 10 samples of snuff preserved in metallic wrappings; in 3 samples, where the wrapping was made of lead, he found that the tobacco closest to the wrapping contained 0.76:100 of lead, and the tobacco in the center of the packet contained 0.31:100. *Schutzenberg* and *Boutmy*, in food preserves intended for the navy, found lead stemming from the tinning of the containers, in amounts varying from 4.5 to 948 milligrams per can. The same can be said for sweet pastes colored with lead chromate; *Denison Stewart* reported a case where eight people died in convulsions after eating a cake colored with chrome yellow; in some confections colored with chrome yellow instead of egg yellow, *Galippe* noted that the paste contained 0.060 per 100 of metallic lead. The practice of clarifying wine and other alcoholic beverages with Saturn's salt can make them toxic, as can their more or less prolonged containment in lead vessels, in pottery, or in glasses whose glaze is based on this metal. Water, too, can become impregnated with lead from pumps, containers, taps, lead pipes, or coated with lead-based paint.

Accidental poisonings can still be observed from the use of food substances wrapped in coarse papers, deceitfully made heavier by the addition of lead, or of powders, makeup, made with white lead or red lead, of hair dyes based on Saturn's salt. *Lemaistre* observed an epidemic of saturnism, due to a millstone, which had been repaired with lead; the flour from it contained 3 milligrams of the metal per kilogram.

Intoxication can also be caused by simply staying in rooms painted with white lead, basic lead carbonate, or other lead-based colors.

Troisier asserts that the type of coal known as "chemical braise" can produce lead poisoning, containing up to 6:100 of lead nitrate; even the dust raised by this coal contains a considerable amount of lead.

Ritter confirmed the poisoning of five people who had eaten hare preserved for three days in a mixture of wine and vinegar. He was able to extract 17 lead shots from the body of the animal. Chemical analysis of the leftovers from the meal and of the vomited substances revealed the presence of this metal. Also, the common practice of using lead shot to clean bottles is dangerous; often some shots remain stuck to the bottom of the bottle and can poison the wine that is introduced into it.

Acute poisoning (*Acute Saturnism*). - It is usually caused by the ingestion of a soluble lead compound (mostly lead acetate) or of some substance accidentally mixed with a more or less significant quantity of lead.

Symptoms of acute poisoning. – At the moment of ingestion, a sweetish, astringent, metallic taste in the mouth and a constriction in the throat is felt. Soon the symptoms of intense gastroenteritis appear: sharp pains localized at first in the epigastrium and then spreading throughout the abdomen, nausea followed sometimes by vomiting, constipation or diarrhea, burning thirst, weak and frequent pulse, oliguria, and nervous symptoms: trembling of the limbs, general prostration, coma, death in a few hours or days. In other cases, after a period of debilitation and mild nervous symptoms, recovery occurs very slowly.

Treatment. – In recent cases, gastric lavage, emetics, laxatives. The antidotes are alkaline sulfates (sodium sulfate, magnesium sulfate) that form insoluble lead sulfate, albumin, milk.

Chronic Poisoning (*Chronic Lead Poisoning*). – Occupational poisoning is most frequently observed among workers who extract lead in mines, or who process this metal, manufacturers and grinders of pigments (red lead, white lead, chrome yellow, massicot yellow, chrome green), mirror cleaners, cartridge makers, painters and decorators of apartments, varnish producers, founders, gas workers, typographers, print character cleaners, in tinsmiths, enamelers, pottery workers, etc. Other times, the cause of intoxication is not so easy to find. Fouque reported a case of chronic lead poisoning in a hunter who habitually kept a shotgun pellet in his mouth, to always have it ready in any event where he had to quickly reload his weapon; *Bourguet* in a fisherman, who used to hold a series of lead pellets in his mouth through a wire, to be able to unwind the line properly and cast it into the water with skill. *Fornaca* observed a case of chronic lead poisoning with severe colic for 16 years, bilateral radial paralysis in a saddler who for twenty years used a newspaper instead of a tablecloth, and on top of it arranged his food; such a fact should not surprise, when one considers that newspaper ink contains lead.

Symptoms of Chronic Poisoning. - They can appear after a few days, but usually develop after two or more months of stay in an environment tainted by lead emissions, or contact with lead, and can be divided into general symptoms and special symptoms. The former are those that characterize the so-called saturnine cachexia: a bluish or slate-gray coloration of the portion of the gum closest to the tooth, which is blackish at its base (lead sulfide); sweet and astringent taste in the mouth, fetid breath, saturnine jaundice, general and more pronounced emaciation in the face, serious muscular and nervous weakness, etc. This cachexia frequently leads in women to metrorrhagia and abortions; *Roque,* moreover, in a series of observations collected at the "Salpêtrière" and "Bicêtre", has noted numerous cases of idiocy, imbecility, epilepsy, in children born from lead-afflicted parents.

We then have another series of symptoms, due to the specific professions practiced by the patients, and even more so to their individual predisposition. Such phenomena can be classified into five distinct groups: saturnine colic - anesthesia - paralysis - arthralgia - encephalopathy, although in the same individual, phenomena belonging to two or several of these various groups often manifest simultaneously or successively.

a) **Saturnine Colic** (*Lead Colic, Painter's Colic*). - It is the most common and earliest manifestation of chronic lead poisoning, and is characterized by intense, constrictive pain in the umbilical region (rarely in the hypogastrium or any other point of the abdomen), relieved by pressure (patients lie on their stomach, pressing it with their hands). There is also nausea and vomiting, obstinate constipation, dyspnea, slowing of the pulse at the height of the attack; the abdomen is hard and contracted.

These colic attacks last from a few minutes to over an hour, may recur several times in a single day, and for several consecutive days.

They can also stop spontaneously, and the patient regains, at least for some time, his relative health. Only exceptionally can saturnine colic, without other complications, be fatal.

b) **Saturnine Anesthesia** - This condition is also very frequently encountered in chronic lead poisoning. It may be limited to the skin (of the trunk and limbs) or to the muscles; it generally follows motor paralysis. Other times it affects the sensory organs, hence more or less complete blindness, hearing disturbances, more rarely taste and smell.

c) **Saturnine Paralysis** - In most cases, it follows saturnine colic or some other manifestation of lead poisoning. It preferentially affects the extensor muscles of the hand on the forearm, and sometimes also the biceps, deltoid, and long supinator, very rarely the muscles of the lower limbs. It may also affect the trunk muscles and respiratory muscles, with a rapidly fatal outcome. It is rarely associated with cutaneous anesthesia and is generally bilateral.

d) **Saturnine Arthralgia** - It is characterized by dull and deep, or sharp and piercing pains in the joints of the lower limbs (hip, knee) or upper limbs (armpit, elbow), more rarely in other joints, without any symptoms of inflammation. These pains occur in ordinarily nocturnal attacks and may also be located in the skin, bones, or muscles.

e) **Saturnine Encephalopathy.** - Of the various saturnine manifestations, this is undoubtedly the most serious. It generally constitutes the final scene of intoxication but may also be found at the beginning of the disease. The severe cerebral symptoms manifest (sometimes preceded by dizziness, headache, slight tremors of the arms and hands) with furious or melancholic delirium, convulsions sometimes associated with loss of consciousness, and in some cases simulating attacks of tetanus or epilepsy, sopor or coma.

Furthermore, amblyopia or amaurosis may be observed; in severe cases, the outcome can be fatal.

Anatomical Lesions. - Almost always the necroscopic finding is negative; in certain cases, lead was found in the nervous centers and nerves; the muscles may appear atrophic and in fatty degeneration, the kidneys may present epithelial desquamation of the tubules or also appear in fatty degeneration.

Treatment of Chronic Lead Poisoning. - Good ventilation of workshops and factories, scrupulous body cleanliness (baths), long rests in the open air, frequent use of purgatives, and a strengthening diet constitute the best prophylactic means.

Baths and general massage are the most suitable means

to promote the elimination of lead from the body. According to *Dixon Mann*, potassium iodide does not favor the elimination of the metal, although it may still be useful in lead poisoning due to other actions. *Peyron* praises the good effects of sodium sulfide (at a dose of 0.30-0.50), and according to *Quinquand*, this salt not only favors the elimination of lead but also that of mercury, which is why he believes this medication can be usefully administered in all forms of metal poisoning. *Semmola* recommends the use of direct current, advising to apply the positive pole to the tongue and the negative to the epigastrium every morning for 10-15 minutes, and then to run the positive pole along the sides of the spinal column and the negative on the abdomen.

For colics, to calm the pains, recourse to atropine and opium will be made; *Combemale* affirms that high doses of olive oil (200 grams, first producing tolerance on the part of the stomach with cocaine, menthol, etc.) have a decongestant and sedative action in saturnine colic superior to that of any other drug. In cases of paralysis, baths, massage, electrotherapy, and strychnine will be beneficial. In the treatment of saturnine encephalopathy, the use of potassium iodide combined with bromide generally gives the best results. Martial preparations, quinine, strychnine are to be prescribed in cases of great weakness or notable cachexia.

Copper (Cu.).

Metallic copper is not poisonous. A prominent Russian

physiologist, *Pélikan*, boiled food in copper vessels, then measured with chemical analysis the amount of copper that these foods might contain, and found only insignificant traces of the metal. Therefore, he believes that such foods can never cause intoxication. Nowadays, it is universally acknowledged that copper vessels are much less dangerous than those tinned with lead-bearing tin; it is also known that the sacred vessels of the Jews were made of copper, and that Moses, who was not only a great legislator but also, relatively to his times, a notable hygienist, had prescribed no other standard for these vessels than meticulous cleanliness. However, this harmlessness does not extend to copper salts; they can indeed be causes of poisoning, although very rarely, because copper salts are not absorbed by the mucosa of the digestive tract unless it has been cauterized, and such cauterization does not occur with small or moderate doses, and large doses are readily detected because of their extremely unpleasant taste. Moreover, cupric salts are vigorous emetics, so in the vast majority of cases the poison is expelled before its harmful action on the organism has time to manifest. As early as 1877, *Pasteur* had acknowledged that the use of vegetables greened with copper posed no danger; *Du Moulin* consumed for himself and his family, for fourteen months, bread to which a small amount of copper sulfate had been added to make it whiter and softer, without observing any sort of disturbances..

Acute poisoning. –Cupric intoxication can be caused by the use of fatty or acidic foods cooked and allowed to cool in copper, brass, or bronze containers, in which a sometimes considerable quantity of copper oxide (verdigris) can be found. The same oxide can form from the storage of alcoholic beverages (wine, beer, etc.) in copper vessels. Typically, however, it is due to the ingestion of copper salts in solution, copper acetate (green vitriol or copperas) and especially copper sulfate (blue vitriol, blue copperas), which is the most active.

Symptoms. - Almost immediately after ingestion there is a disgusting, astringent taste in the mouth, with nausea and persistent vomiting, ptyalism. Soon, excruciating colicky pains and diarrhea with very frequent bowel movements, sometimes bloody, ensue. From the nervous system, headaches, dizziness, and in severe cases anesthesia, paralysis, delirium, collapse are observed. If the poisoning is caused by the ingestion of foods cooked and preserved in copper containers, the symptoms manifest 8-15 hours after the meal.

Anatomical lesions. - They are not constant; sometimes, in addition to signs of inflammation, the gastroenteric mucosa may present erosions, ulcerations, or disseminated gangrenous patches; ecchymoses have been found in the submucosal cellular tissue. In very rare cases, subpericardial, subperitoneal, or subpleural hemorrhages are noted. Rarely does the digestive tract show, throughout its length, any trace of irritation or inflammation.

Treatment. - In recent cases, clear the stomach with a gastric pump, with emetics. Burnt magnesia, egg white water, milk, iron sulfate, iron hydrate or filings, wood charcoal powder are generally used remedies to neutralize the poison.

Anti-inflammatory, antispasmodic, narcotic, etc., agents will be beneficial in combating the various symptoms.

Chronic Poisoning. - It is doubtful whether true chronic copper poisoning exists; many completely deny it. Copper is not a poison that accumulates (like lead) in the body to manifest itself after a longer or shorter period; numerous observations made on workers who handle this metal and on those who prepare verdigris and cartridge cases for ammunition have allowed us to note that these workers do not suffer from any particular disease related to their occupation. More likely, the symptoms attributed to copper colic are simply the result of fatigue and the heat that overcomes these workers (*Du Moulin*). There is rather a sort of impregnation; in foundries, in workshops where copper is handled, there are workers who are impregnated with the metal, with teeth, hair, and beards of an indelible greenish tint, yet they enjoy enviable health.

In the village of Durfort an entire industrial population (coppersmiths, copper beaters) lives for twelve hours a day in an environment saturated with copper dust, without showing any particular morbid phenomenon, nor is the average mortality rate higher than that of other agricultural populations in the region.

When colics and cachexia do occur, it is lead, zinc, arsenic, metals so often mixed with copper, that must be blamed (*Toussaint*).

Zinc (Zn).

Zinc compounds act on the body like those of copper, however, their toxicity is much less, except for zinc chloride ($ZnCl_2$) which possesses very strong caustic properties.

In zinc chloride poisoning, symptoms of severe gastroenteritis are noted, with violent vomiting, very frequent bowel evacuations, intense colic, sharp pain in the epigastric region, and albuminuria. In severe cases, intense dyspnea, symptoms of collapse; death occurs due to cardiac paralysis, preceded by respiratory arrest. Autopsy findings include the mucosa of the mouth being white and opaque, that of the stomach sometimes tough and leather-like, sometimes wrinkled, opaque, and of a dark leaden color; in addition, congestion of the kidneys and lungs is observed.

For treatment, recourse will be had to tannin, albumin water, and alkaline carbonates.

Mercury (Hg).

When ingested in large amounts (100-200 grams), metallic mercury quickly passes through the gastro-enteric tract, usually without causing severe disturbances; in moderate doses, however, it is partially absorbed from the intestine and may over time present symptoms of intoxication. Cases of poisoning by mercurial compounds are not so rare, both because of their very common use in therapy as antiseptics and anti-syphilitics, and because of their daily use in a multitude of industries. The toxicity of these compounds is also well known to the public, which sufficiently explains the numerous cases of accidental, criminal, or suicidal poisoning. The soluble mercurial preparations (corrosive sublimate, mercuric iodide, mercuric nitrate) are the most dangerous; but also of the insoluble ones (metallic mercury, red sulfide or cinnabar, black sulfide, calomel, mercurous iodide), some, by transforming more or less slowly in the body, likewise give rise to poisoning.

Acute Poisoning (Acute Hydrargyrism) - When a soluble mercurial compound (mostly corrosive sublimate) is ingested in high doses, a violent gastroenteritis with severe nervous disorders ensues. The symptoms, primarily observed in such cases, include burning, excruciating pain in the mouth, pharynx, esophagus, and especially in the stomach and intestines, sometimes bloody vomiting, bloody diarrhea accompanied by extremely painful tenesmus, oliguria or anuria, prostration, fainting spells, cutaneous anesthesia, collapse. Death, due to cardiac paralysis, can occur within half an hour, but usually happens after 24-36 hours. In milder cases, when the dose of the ingested poison is smaller, there are symptoms of toxic gastroenteritis with albuminuria, which often ends with recovery.

Anatomical Lesions. - The gastroenteric mucosa is swollen, red, softened, and sometimes gangrenous here and there. The intestinal mucosa shows ecchymoses along its entire length, which are also found in the mesentery. *Taylor* saw a case with stomach perforation. The renal parenchyma is intensely injected, especially at the level of the Malpighian glomeruli; the kidney is in a granular-fatty state identical to that seen in poisoning by caustic acids, ammonia, arsenic, phosphorus. There is also congestion of the trachea and bronchi and pinpoint ecchymoses under the pericardium and under the endocardium. The blood is black and fluid.

Treatment. - The antidotes are albumin, milk, and freshly prepared iron sulfate. Otherwise, the treatment is symptomatic.

Soluble mercury salts, *applied* externally to sores, ulcers, wounds, in the form of powders, pastes, concentrated solutions, locally cause intense inflammation, and 4-8 hours after their application the symptoms of acute poisoning by ingestion occur.

Chronic Mercury Poisoning (Chronic Hydrargyrism). - Workers who extract mercury from mines or obtain mercury from ores, and those in professions requiring the use of mercury (gilders, mirror silverers, barometer and thermometer makers, etc.) exhibit specific afflictions, among which are primarily mercurial stomatitis and mercurial tremor.

Mercurial Stomatitis. - The oral mucosa is covered with a purulent, greasy plaster; the gums are swollen, red, detached, and easily bleed.

There is also noted ptyalism (up to 5 liters of saliva in 24 hours), swelling of the salivary glands and adjacent lymphatic glands, extremely foul breath, and subjective symptoms: difficulty or inability to speak and swallow, insomnia; sometimes death ensues with terrible suffering, as observed on the ship "The

Triumph" where nearly all crew members, by inhaling mercury vapors leaking from the barrels transported by the ship, were struck by such intense stomatitis that two of them died.

Ptyalism may occur without stomatitis, as this inflammation may also occur without a noticeable increase in salivary secretion. Stomatitis may be preceded or accompanied by general symptoms: severe weakness, anorexia, nausea, vomiting, bloody stools or even constipation, fever (*mercurial fever*), and is also frequently observed in individuals undergoing mercurial treatments.

Moutard-Martin observed cases of mercurialism in people living near a laboratory where mercury was used.

Mercurial Tremor. - Workers handling mercury are often affected by a particular tremor of the limbs, which usually starts slowly and is typically preceded by headaches, dizziness, psychological excitation (*mercurial erethism*) so that the slightest surprise, the least emotion, the mere presence of a doctor is enough to induce a choreiform agitation in their limbs (*Hammond*).

The tremor almost always begins in the hands and arms, and later the lower limbs are affected, making the gait wobbly and uncertain, to the point of confining the severely afflicted to bed in serious cases.

The muscles of the tongue also show disordered contractions, making speech difficult and stuttering. This tremor is intentional, meaning it does not exist when the body is at rest; psychological excitations (anger, fright, etc.) exacerbate it; at other times it is influenced by other causes.

Thus, *Fourcroy* recounts that a drunken gilder could, in a state of intoxication, hold a glass and bring it steadily to his lips, something he could not do when sober.

In individuals who continue to be exposed to mercury vapors, the tremor is subsequently accompanied by painful cramps, localized paralysis often in the lower extremities, and often also extending to all limb muscles. *Adder* observed in a very advanced case also paralysis of the muscles of swallowing and mastication. In addition, disturbances of intelligence or even severe neuropathies (epilepsy, dementia, etc.) arise.

In addition to stomatitis and tremor, a severe cachexia is not uncommon in hydrargyrism, characterized by nervous exhaustion, profound anemia, progressive weight loss up to the most marked marasmus, earthy-yellow complexion, and skin ulcers. In other cases, there is a peculiar predisposition to suffer from gastroenteritis, pulmonary tuberculosis, chronic nephritis, etc.; in women, miscarriage is very common.

Anatomical Lesions. -Fatty degeneration of organs and sometimes deposits of calcium salts in the kidneys; brittle, decalcified bones. In the cadavers of cachectic individuals, fatty degeneration of the myocardium and liver, kidneys, spleen, and intestinal vessels is often found.

Treatment. - Prompt removal of the patient from the sources of poisoning; nutritious diet, potassium iodide, hyoscine, sometimes also galvanization. Against stomatitis and ptyalism, atropine, potassium chlorate mouthwashes. Treatment of various symptoms.

Antimony (Sb).

Antimonial poisoning is rare; it generally concerns the untimely administration of tartar emetic to tender children or even to adults, due to a pronounced idiosyncrasy to this medication. Other times, the poisoning is intentional or criminal; Tardieu saw tartar emetic used as an abortive substance in a case that proved fatal.

Tartar emetic $C^4H^4O^6K(SbO)$ is a white substance, consisting of tetrahedral or octahedral crystals; it dissolves in 25 parts of cold water and in 2 parts of hot water; the solution has a slightly metallic and sugary taste.

Symptoms of poisoning. - At the time of ingestion, a metallic taste is felt in the mouth, and soon after, the symptoms of a violent gastroenteritis appear (repeated, copious, and stubborn vomiting, diarrheal discharges, sharp pain in the epigastrium, oliguria) with nervous disturbances: agitation, fainting, prostration, dizziness. Around the fourth or fifth day, a pustular rash appears on the skin of the limbs and on various other parts of the body. The symptoms worsen, hiccups, delirium, anuria, convulsions, collapse ensue; death in 2-6 days, in children within a few hours.

In rarer cases, death from collapse and paralysis occurs before the symptoms of toxic gastroenteritis have had time to manifest.

Ordinarily, however, the abundance and rapidity with which vomiting occurs, opposing the absorption of the toxin, as well as the promptness and effectiveness of the treatment, save the patient from death; a gradual improvement of symptoms is noted, with recovery in 8–15 days.

Anatomical lesions. - The gastroenteric mucosa is strongly inflamed, softened; it often may show scattered reddish-brown patches or pustules in the region of the pharynx, esophagus, and stomach. The inner surface of the stomach is in some cases covered with a dense, blackish, sometimes bloody coating; spleen swollen; liver in fatty degeneration (*Grohe* and *Mosler* from Greinfswald reported that the countrywomen of the Duchy of Brunswick, who trade in fat geese, introduce a certain quantity of white antimony oxide into the feeding of these animals). The lungs often appear congested, as well as the brain and the cranial meninges.

Treatment. - Empty the stomach with a gastric pump, also resorting to emetics (copper or zinc sulfate, etc.) when vomiting has ceased too soon. The antidotes are tannic preparations (walnut husk decoction, rhatany extract, cinchona decoction, etc.) and especially tannic acid in substance.

Beneficial are also calcined magnesia, alkaline sulphides, stimulants (coffee, ether, etc.). During convalescence, light feeding, a milk diet is recommended.

Applied externally over ulcers, sores, wounds, tartar emetic is also easily absorbed by the body, and besides the local symptoms of irritation, it can cause sometimes fatal poisoning. *Tardieu* reports the case of a woman who applied to a small breast sore a salve given by a charlatan and died within a few hours. Chemical analysis showed the salve to be made up in equal parts of lard and tartar emetic.

Chronic poisoning. - Following the repeated and prolonged administration of tartar emetic, nausea, vomiting, prostration, diarrhea alternating with constipation, severe muscular weakness, fainting, pustular skin rash are observed.

The course of the disease is very slow, with remissions and exacerbations that may or may not occur close together; it can last several months, and death ensues due to the progressive wasting away of the body, sometimes preceded by convulsions.

Treatment. - Tannic preparations; symptomatic care.

Potassium Nitrate (Nitre, saltpeter, KNO_3)

This salt is found naturally on the surface of the soil, on old walls. In Peru, there are large deposits known as "caliche or nitre earth," varying in thickness from 0.3 to 1.5 meters, and spanning over thirty miles near Copiago, in northern Chile. It is a white substance that crystallizes in hexagonal prisms, soluble in water, insoluble in pure alcohol, with a taste that is initially refreshing, then pungent, salty, and bitter. It is widely used in the manufacture of gunpowder, nitric acid, and other chemical compounds; it also serves to preserve meats. It was often mistaken for Epsom or Glauber's salt, thus leading to accidental poisonings. The lethal dose would be 34 grams, but according to *Orfila*, 8-12 grams taken at once could suffice.

Symptoms of poisoning. - A quarter of an hour or half an hour after ingestion, there is an internal sensation of cold with bilious or bloody vomiting, copious, similarly bloody diarrhea, intense abdominal and gastric pain. Symptoms of general and profound collapse appear rapidly: cold skin, very weak pulse, muscle cramps, dizziness, fainting, convulsions, and coma. Death usually occurs within a few hours (2-5), rarely after 2-3 days.

Anatomical lesions. - The gastric mucosa is reddened, with small black spots scattered here and there, sometimes eroded, rarely ulcerated. The stomach may be filled with non-coagulated blood. The blood is fluid, of a bright vermillion color.

The *treatment* is symptomatic: pieces of ice, stimulants (camphor, ether), narcotics (opium).

II - Irritant Vegetable Poisons.

Croton oil plant (Croton tiglium, L.).

This euphorbiaceous plant is a shrub that grows in the Moluccas Islands. The seeds, the only part used of the plant, are ovoid, elongated, slightly angular, blunt at both ends, covered with a yellowish epidermis spotted with brown marks. The face bearing the hilum shows several longitudinal veins; the lateral veins are more prominent and form bumps near the base of the seed.

These seeds, when pressed, yield a yellow or reddish oil with an unpleasant odor and a sharp and burning taste; it is one of the most violent drastic poisons; 6 drops of this oil, in a case reported by *Widal*, were a lethal dose for a forty-year-old man.

According to *Buchheim*, the active principle of croton oil is an acid, which he named crotonoleic acid.

Symptoms of poisoning. - Some time after ingestion, intense toxic gastroenteritis manifests, with violent and repeated vomiting, profuse serous and bloody diarrhea, burning pains in the throat and stomach, excruciating colic, sometimes muscle cramps, and final collapse.

In some cases, symptoms of gastroenteritis are absent, and death occurs within a few hours (4-24) due to paralysis of the nervous system.

Treatment. - It is necessary to empty the stomach with a gastric pump and emetics, administer plenty of milk, mucilaginous drinks, opiates, and hot baths. Ammonia, brandy, and other stimulants will be used against collapse.

Colocynth (*Cucumis colocynthis*).

This cucurbitaceous plant has alternate, sharp, 5-lobed leaves, large yellow monopetal flowers with 5 divisions; the fruit is globular, yellow, the size of an orange, smooth, covered with a hard, leathery, thin rind enclosing a white and spongy pulp in which numerous seeds

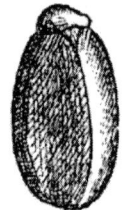

are found. It is indigenous to the East and the islands of the Archipelago; the colocynth of commerce is the fruit stripped of its envelope, and it appears in whitish, light, dry, spongy masses of extraordinarily bitter taste.

6 centigrams of colocynth already provoke profuse diarrhea; higher doses can cause colic, bloody diarrhea, nausea, and vomiting with intense inflammation of the gastroenteric mucosa. 5 grams can be a lethal dose.

The treatment is identical to that for croton oil poisoning.

Colchicum (*Colchicum autumnale*, L.).

The bulb of the colchicum is solid and fleshy, irregularly ovoid, compressed on one side, where it presents a deep longitudinal groove due to the presence of the stem. The flowers are very large, of a pale violet color, consisting of a long tube 22–23 centimeters in length, with a bell-shaped limb, with 6 deep divisions, appearing in the month of September, long before the leaves, which do not develop until the following spring, along with the fruits. This plant, belonging to the lily family, is common in damp pastures, mainly in the regions of the Mediterranean and Central Europe. All parts of the plant, but especially the bulb and seeds, are poisonous.

The alkaloid is colchicine ($C_{22}H_{25}NO^6$), a very active substance, since a dose of 4 centigrams can be fatal to a man; however, poisoning is quite rare..

Symptoms of poisoning. - These are those of severe gastroenteritis with violent vomiting, profuse and bloody diarrhea; burning pain in the throat and stomach. Additionally, there are headaches, dyspnea, weak and very small pulse; severe prostration, a drop in temperature. Consciousness remains unaltered; death occurs due to general paralysis, sometimes preceded by spasms and convulsions.

In a case of fatal poisoning observed by *Odermatt*, there were vomiting, significant frequency of pulse and respiration, dilated pupils, sluggish and then rigid, conjunctivitis, strabismus, 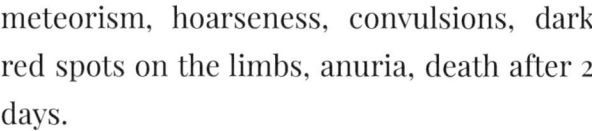 meteorism, hoarseness, convulsions, dark red spots on the limbs, anuria, death after 2 days.

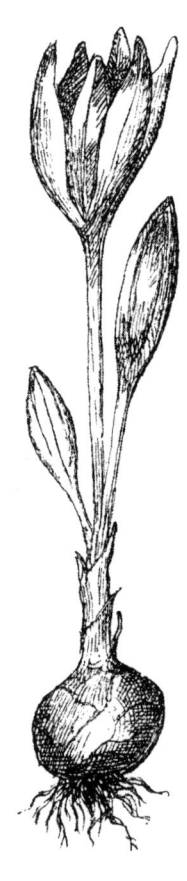

Anatomical lesions. - In addition to signs of violent inflammation of the gastro-enteric mucosa, the lungs, liver, kidneys, brain are congested, and sometimes the spinal cord is inflamed (*Warncke*).

Treatment. - Emetics, stomach pump. The antidotes are tannic acid and iodine water. To alleviate the inflammation of the digestive tract, milk, oily and mucilaginous drinks, opiates will be administered. Ether injections against prostration and collapse.

White Hellebore
(*Veratrum album*, L.).

This plant, belonging to the lily family, grows in high Alpine pastures; it has a fleshy, taproot, a straight, striated stem about 65 centimeters high, ending in a panicle of greenish flowers; its leaves are sessile, oval, sharp, marked by longitudinal folds.

The active principle is veratrine ($C^{32}H^{52}N^{2}O^{8}$), which acts on the body in a way similar to colchicine. Cases of poisoning have also been noted due to the accidental or criminal mixing of veratrine powder in snuff tobacco.

The treatment consists of administering tannin, opiates, stimulants (coffee, alcohol, etc.) and skin revulsives.

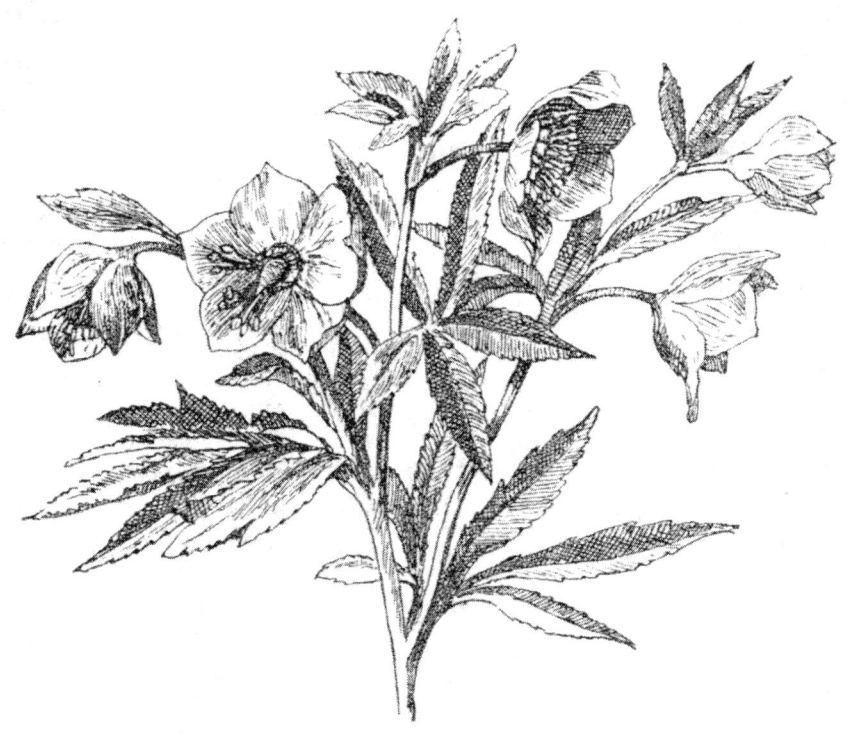

Sabina (*Juniperus sabina*, L.).

This conifer grows in high, arid, and stony places; it has a trunk ranging from 4 to 4.5 meters in height, extremely small leaves that are squamiform, straight, close-set, opposite, sharp, dioecious flowers, and pisiform, ovoid, fleshy fruits of a bluish-black color containing one or two small seeds.

The leaves, especially, have an irritating action when administered in powder or infusion, due to the essential oil (terpineol) they contain. In most cases, sabina is used by the common folk to induce abortion, and not infrequently results in fatal poisonings.

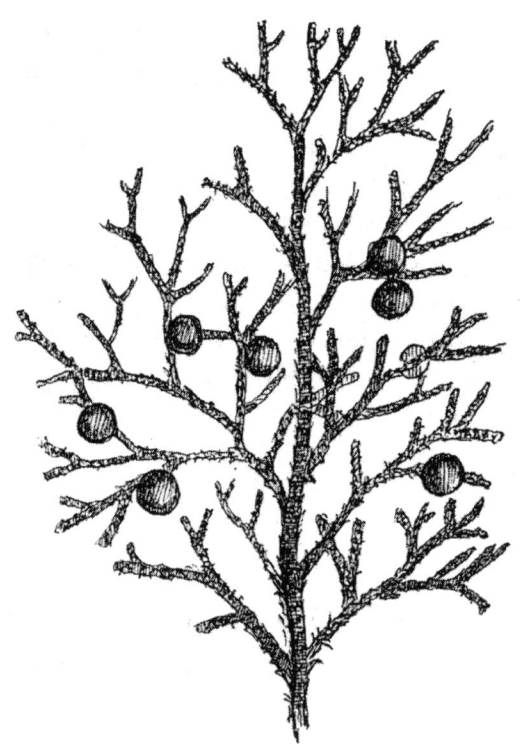

Symptoms of poisoning. - Following the ingestion of sabina preparations, signs of severe inflammation of the digestive tract with repeated vomiting, profuse diarrhea, and intense colicky pain appear after some time. Also noted are fever, hemorrhages (epistaxis, hematuria, metrorrhagia, etc.), ptyalism, strangury, and in certain cases collapse and death. Other times the fatal outcome occurs in complete insensibility, and is preceded by convulsions. In pregnant women, abortion is not rare, with the expulsion of a dead or dying fetus.

Anatomical lesions. - At autopsy, inflammation of the stomach, intestines, and kidneys, congestion of the liver are found. *Murray* found in one case the gallbladder ruptured. Signs of peritonitis are not rare.

Treatment. - Emetics, gastric lavage; symptomatic care.

Poisonous Mushrooms.

Among the mushrooms of the genus "Amanita," which are usually edible and highly sought after for their delicacy, there are some highly poisonous species, especially the false golden amanita (amanita muscaria or agaricus pseudo-aurantiacus), the venomous amanita, the verrucosa, the amanita phalloides.

The amanita muscaria or false fly agaric, which is the most common and frequent cause of mushroom poisoning, has a globular, convex cap covered with a reddish-orange film, in turn covered by the volva regularly divided into white or yellowish-

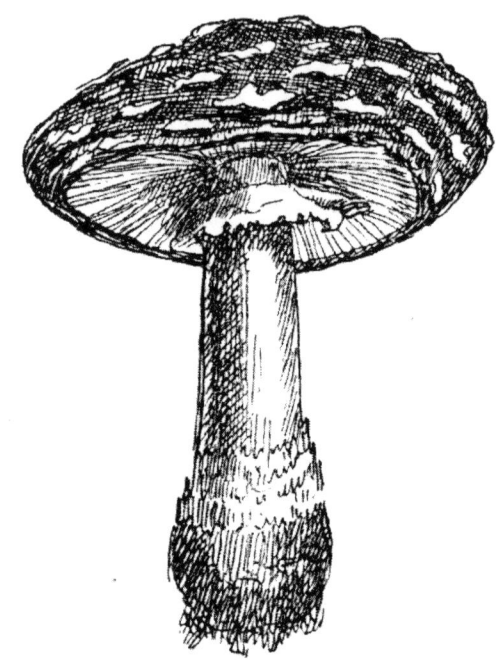

orange warts. Its flesh is white but stained yellow beneath the film. The stem is firm, somewhat bulbous at the top, white and hairy; the volva's base is attached to the bulb, often leaving a collar made up of several layers of concentric scales. *Schmideberg* and *Koppe* isolated from this mushroom an alkaloid they called muscarine ($C^5H^{13}NO^2$), a substance that crystallizes in plates, odorless, tasteless, soluble in water; heated to 100° it emits an odor reminiscent of tobacco; it can be obtained chemically by the oxidation of choline. Amanitin is another toxic principle extracted by *Letellier*; it is a liquid with an unpleasant smell, volatile; heated with nitric acid it transforms into muscarine.

In addition to the mushrooms of the genus amanita, the venomous agaric (agaricus necator), the emetic agaric (ag. pectinatus), the bloody agaric (ag. sanguineus), the Medusa head agaric (ag. annularius), the styptic agaric (ag. stypticus), the pernicious bolete (boletus luridus) and many others are also poisonous and are too often confused with the harmless species.

However, it should not be forgotten that even edible mushrooms, if spoiled or putrefied, acquire toxic qualities, and that those that are fresh and healthy, if ingested in large amounts, can often cause violent and severe indigestion, such as to simulate poisoning.

Symptoms and course of poisoning. - A few hours after the ingestion of the mushrooms, and in some cases the following day, the symptoms of intoxication begin, which sometimes simply manifest with dizziness, stupor, severe general weakness, and visual disturbances (objects appear tinged with blue), without any gastric symptom.

However, in most cases, there are nausea, abundant, repeated, obstinate vomiting, sometimes bloody diarrhea, tenesmus, and intense colicky pain, a feeling of constriction in the throat with intense thirst and ptyalism.

In addition to the symptoms of toxic gastroenteritis, there are usually nervous disorders, heaviness of the head, headache, dizziness, stupor. The pulse is weak and rapid, the pupils are constricted, the urine is scarce, containing hemoglobin, or even suppressed; the patients are comatose; in certain cases delirium, hallucinations, mania, cramps, and tetanic or epileptic convulsions occur; sometimes jaundice manifests. Death can occur within two or three days with symptoms of profound collapse or amid convulsions.

Anatomical lesions. - In addition to signs of inflammation, ecchymotic or gangrenous patches can sometimes be found scattered on the mucosa of the stomach and intestines. The liver is ordinarily enlarged, softened, in fatty degeneration, which is also observed in the stomach and kidneys. The spleen often appears swollen and congested.

Treatment. - Prevention mainly consists in disseminating, especially in countries where there is a high consumption of mushrooms, the knowledge necessary to distinguish suspicious from harmless fungi. Therefore, schools will be equipped with large wall charts, or even better, models representing the various species of mushrooms in their natural state, pointing out to students the necessity of relying only on those whose harmlessness they can certainly recognize. In cities, active surveillance of markets by knowledgeable individuals is essential, and the same vigilance must be exercised over the preparation and sale of dried and preserved mushrooms.

The treatment consists in the administration of emetics and purgatives. The antidote, or rather the antagonist, of muscarine is atropine. The beneficial action of this alkaloid in muscarine poisoning is significant and certain, even in the more advanced stages of poisoning, and only fails when circulation and respiration are on the verge of cessation. *Königsdorfer* claims to have achieved remarkable and sometimes instantaneous successes with hypodermic injections of strychnine at a dose of 1 milligram at a time (maximum total dose: 12 milligrams).

Stimulants (coffee, ether, etc.) and opiates are also very useful.

III – Irritant Animal Poisons

Putrefied Meat

Putrefied meat, and perhaps even that from animals that have died of disease, is dangerous, and its consumption frequently leads to severe, often fatal, intoxications. Experiments by *Selmi, Guareschi, Brieger,* and others have shown that a large number of ptomaines (diamines belonging to the fatty series, nitrogenous bases like the vegetable alkaloids) are produced in the putrefaction of meat, many of which have considerable toxicity; among these are noted hydrocollidine ($C^8H^{13}N$), a convulsant poison; gadinine ($C^7H^{18}N^2O^6$); parvoline ($C^{17}H^{36}N^4$). It has also been observed that these toxic alkaloids develop especially when the meat, having been deprived of air exposure for a longer or shorter period, is subsequently exposed to oxygen; this at least explains the numerous cases of poisoning from the consumption of meat contained in cans that have been open for several days. It is also worth noting that cooking does not always completely destroy these poisonous substances.

A frequent cause of intoxication from spoiled meat is due to the habit, common among gourmets, especially when it comes to game, of not eating it unless it is already in a state of putrefaction, regardless of the serious risks they take to satisfy their, in some respects, questionable gluttony. Poisonings from the consumption of spoiled sausages, which especially in Germany and the Netherlands take the form of veritable epidemics, are also frequent; this is not surprising, considering the large consumption by the less affluent classes, which are also the most numerous, and the difficulty in recognizing the nature and quality of the substances they contain from their outward appearance. Greedy and unscrupulous traders, who do not hesitate to profit at the expense of their customers' health, boil all the remnants of meat, often already putrefied, at their disposal, finely mince it, season it with many drugs to better mask their repugnant odor and taste, stuff it into casings, make sausages and salamis, which they then sell cheaply and on busy days. The intoxication caused by the consumption of these altered meats was called botulism, from the word "botellus," meaning sausage.

Symptoms of poisoning. - These can be very varied, but some can be considered characteristic. Several hours after ingestion, a violent toxic gastroenteritis with nausea, vomiting sometimes of food, sometimes of bilious substances, intense colic, violent diarrhea, and sometimes bloody stools manifest.

A severe weakness that can lead to paraplegia, headache; the pulse is small and frequent, or in other cases slowed; in severe cases, death usually occurs in profound collapse. Other times the patient appears to suffer from typhus, with stupor, delirium, fever, hemorrhages, and generally (at least 48 hours after ingestion) skin rashes of a polymorphic nature: hives, spots, roseola, erythema, cutaneous hemorrhages.

The course of the disease is often very prolonged, and relapses are not rare.

Anatomical lesions. - The most common and frequent to be observed are strong injection of the gastroenteric mucosa with more or less extensive hemorrhages, and hemorrhages, especially submucous, in the various organs.

Treatment. - It is purely symptomatic. It is necessary to hasten to evacuate the poison with emetics; with gastric lavage, with purgatives (calomel). Subsequently, oily and mucilaginous lavages, stimulants, etc., will be administered. The diet must be light, and the convalescence monitored.

Fish

It is not uncommon to observe, following the consumption of fish, sporadic cases of poisoning or even true epidemics. Some fish have permanently toxic flesh, but fortunately, these are not found in our waters, or at least not in our markets. Some believe that poisons can form in raw fish when they are salted, but experience has shown that poisoning can also occur through the consumption of cooked, smoked, or otherwise prepared fish. According to *Aurep* , it is a solid toxin, according to Liewental a non-solid toxin; *Motchalow* believes that the poison in fish is a product of the oxidation of olein. *Brieger* demonstrated the presence of various toxic substances in decomposed freshwater and marine fish; mainly parvoline ($C^9H^{13}N$),a convulsive poison, muscarine ($C^5H^{15}NO^3$) very poisonous, and betaine ($C^5H^{11}NO^2$) with an effect similar to curare. However, the nature of these poisons is still far from being precisely known.

As for non-decomposed fish, it can be assumed that these

animals, due to an accidental and perhaps morbid virtue, become capable of producing a toxic substance, a ptomaine or something similar; the abdominal viscera especially would contain the poisonous agent (*Arnould*).

Symptoms of poisoning. - They mostly consist of gastric pains, precordial anxiety, a dryness in the mouth and aphonia, dyspnea, and nervous symptoms: dizziness, headache, amblyopia, and in the most serious cases, muscle paresis and paralysis of the muscles of deglutition, weakness of the heart contractions, choking fits. In other cases, symptoms reminiscent of cholera, ileo-typhus, or arsenic poisoning can be observed.

Stevenson, in a case of poisoning from anchovies, initially noted vomiting, weakness of the pulse, tension in the abdominal walls, mild pain in the gastric region; a few hours later, despite the care given to him, the patient died, and the necroscopic examination revealed pronounced rigidity and cyanosis, diffuse edema, a flow of bloody fluid from the nostrils and ears, hemorrhagic patches on the skin, dark-colored pectoral muscles, and emphysema. The liver was friable and hyperemic, as were the kidneys. The heart and the large vessels were empty of blood, the endocardium showed spots, the stomach contained a hundred grams of a semi-fluid substance.

Four individuals, having eaten the same anchovies, also died a few hours later.

Treatment. - It is symptomatic, identical to that of botulism and poisoning from meat.

Mollusks, shellfish.

Everyone is familiar with the phenomena produced by the ingestion of oysters; one of the most common consequences is urticaria. Other mollusks and crustaceans (crabs, lobsters, sea lice, etc.) at certain times of the year, either, as some want, in connection with sexual functions, or as others claim, because they were collected in impure and polluted waters (sewage drains, etc.), acquire toxic properties. It is a recognized fact in England that mollusks collected in the outer harbors, where the sea is rough, are healthy, while those found in docks, where the water is stagnant, are very harmful. In general, it can be said that animals caught in stagnant and corrupted waters are not suitable for consumption. In 1887, some workers, repairing a wooden vessel in the port of Wilkenshavan, found mollusks along the hull of the boat, which they cooked and ate; many of them became seriously ill, and some died. In the liver of the mytilus edulis (sea louse), *Brieger* found a toxic leucomaine, which he called mytilotoxin ($C^6H^{15}NO^2$).

Symptoms of poisoning. - Ordinarily consist of a sense of constriction in the throat, pain in the muscles and bones, psychological excitement, nausea and vomiting, disturbances of sight and speech. The pupils are dilated, insensitive to light; the pulse is weak, irregular, the temperature drops below normal; various rashes appear on the skin; death can occur within a few hours with symptoms of collapse.

Anatomical lesions. - Are not very characteristic and constant; besides signs of violent enteritis, sometimes an acute splenic tumor can be observed; the liver often shows a particular variegated appearance.

Treatment. - Is analogous to that of poisoning from spoiled meat.

Spoiled Cheese.

As cheeses age, they change significantly in constitution; the casein splits, the fat turns into fatty acids, molds grow and multiply, fly larvae pass the first phase of their existence, the cheese acquires a penetrating smell and a spicy taste much sought after by aficionados. *Wiel* and *Gnehm* speak of gigantic forms of cheese, over a century old, that are passed down from father to son and which, in Swiss families, are only visited on major solemnities and with the respect that we have for the dusty bottles, which with their old age almost guarantee the exquisiteness of the wine. However, toxic substances can also develop in cheese; *Vaughan* discovered one and called it "tyrotoxicon." Here too, we are dealing with alkaloids from the ptomaine family.

Symptoms of poisoning. - Are mostly those of a more or less intense gastroenteritis: nausea, vomiting, enteralgia, profuse diarrhea, a sense of heaviness, oppression in the chest. There are also nervous disorders: intense headache, dizziness, visual disturbances, general prostration.

The *treatment* is no different from that of other food poisonings.

EXCITATORY POISONS

I - Poisons with predominantly cerebral action

Belladonna (*Atropa belladonna*, L.).

Belladonna, belonging to the nightshade family, grows along walls and in old ruins, blooming in June, July, and August. It has a thick and fleshy root, a straight stem ranging from 60 to 120 centimeters in height, velvety, branched, and dichotomous; its leaves are alternate, large, stalked, pointed, and velvety. The flowers are large, solitary, stalked, pendulous, and of a dark red color; they have a bell-shaped calyx with five sharp oval divisions, a regular gamopetalous corolla shaped like an elongated bell, narrowed at the bottom into a short tube, and divided at the top into five equal, blunt, and shallow lobes. The fruit is a round, slightly flattened berry, about the size of a cherry, green in color at first, then red, and finally almost black; it has two chambers containing numerous kidney-shaped seeds. All parts of the plant are poisonous; the fruits are a violent toxin, especially dangerous because they resemble cherries, which have often led children to eat them, and their initially sweet taste does not immediately warn

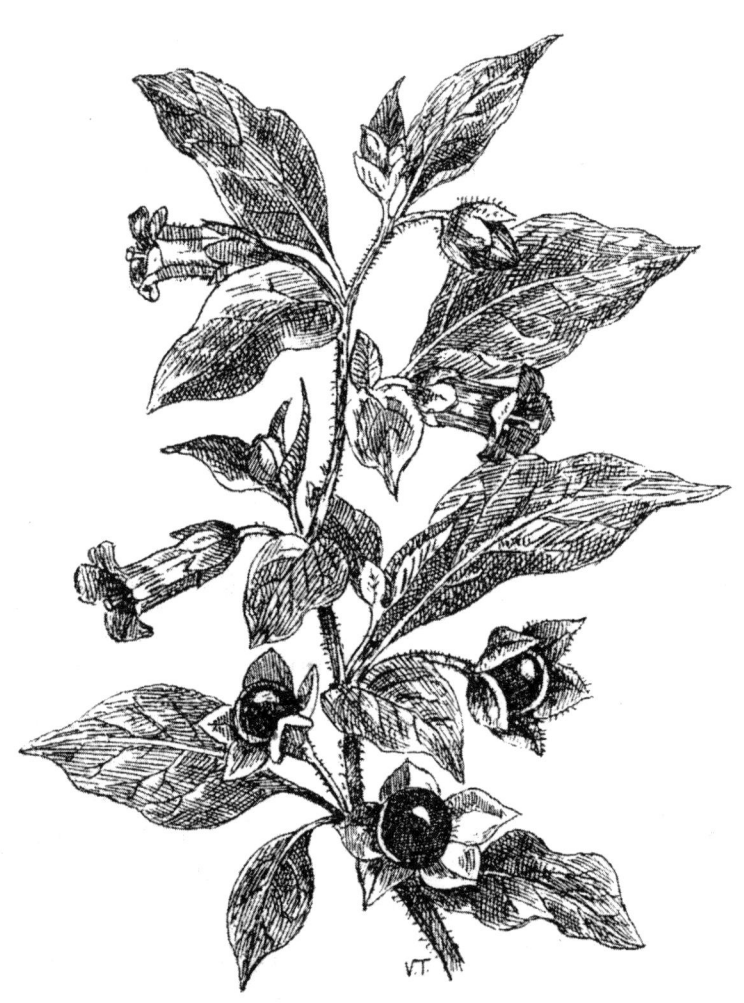

of the danger; the leaves, and above all the root, are endowed with no less energetic and deleterious properties.

Poisoning by belladonna is usually accidental, through ingestion of the fruit or other parts of the plant by children or adults unaware of its poisonous properties, or through the ingestion of pharmaceutical preparations intended for external use, or due to an exaggerated dose. It is known that snails can feed on the leaves of belladonna with impunity, but these mollusks could easily poison those who eat them. Poisoning sometimes occurs from the external use of belladonna plasters or ointments, as in the case observed by *Howart*. It involved a gardener, who, suffering from traumatic lumbago, first rubbed himself with camphorated alcohol, and then applied a belladonna ointment on the skin reddened by these rubbings. In less than three-quarters of an hour, all the symptoms of belladonna poisoning appeared. Even the instillation of overly concentrated solutions of atropine into the eye can be dangerous.

Atropine ($C^{17}H^{25}NO^3$) is the active principle of belladonna. This alkaloid is colorless, odorless, crystallizes in silky, transparent prisms; it is soluble in ether and absolute alcohol, very little in water. It neutralizes acids well, with which it forms easily crystallizable salts. *Kraut* and *Lössen* showed that atropine can split into a volatile base (tropine) and an acid (tropic acid), neither of which have any mydriatic action; *Ladenburg*, by reacting them with each other, was able to synthetically produce atropine. This alkaloid is highly poisonous; 1 decigram is a lethal dose for an adult.

Belladonna, stramonium, henbane, and their alkaloids act

especially on the brain, initially enhancing psychic functions and later paralyzing the brain and peripheral nerves; they also cause slowing of the pulse and a drop in blood pressure.

Symptoms of poisoning. - They usually arise very rapidly and are characterized by a sense of dryness, tightness in the mouth and throat, nausea, and rarely vomiting, dilated pupils with insensitivity to light, blurred vision followed by blindness; staggering gait (patients appear drunk and cannot stand); dizziness followed by fainting; eyes protruding, bloodshot, with a fixed, stupid, or fierce gaze; frequent, small or full, and hard pulse; difficulty breathing; involuntary emission of feces and urine (sphincter paralysis). The skin is hot, intensely itchy, covered with a scarlet fever-like rash. In children, trismus and convulsions are commonly noted; in adults, either cheerful or furious delirium, with hallucinations, followed by coma, convulsions, sometimes a tendency to bite, death from general paralysis in 24-36 hours.

In non-fatal cases, a slow and gradual improvement of symptoms is observed; sometimes fever ensues with profuse sweating, and recovery occurs after 4-8 days.

Poisoning by atropine is not different from that by belladonna except for a quicker course.

Anatomical lesions. - These are neither characteristic nor constant features; they generally consist of intense congestion of the lungs, abdominal viscera, retina, meninges, and brain, associated with hemorrhages: in one case observed by *Rosenberg*, the brain, cerebellum, and medulla oblongata presented numerous foci of capillary hemorrhage.

Treatment. - Emetics, purgatives, stomach pump. The

antidotes to atropine are principally pilocarpine, morphine, and chloral hydrate; morphine is only indicated in the stage of excitement, and not in that of terminal collapse; in this period chloral hydrate may be used, however noting that the heart is further weakened by chloral than by morphine: therefore, stimulants (coffee, alcohol, ether, etc.) and cutaneous revulsives (cold douches on the head, mustard plasters on the chest and calves, etc.) should not be forgotten.

Henbane (*Hyosciamus niger*, L.).

This Solanaceae has an annual root, a stem 45-50 centimeters high, arched and branching in its upper part, covered with long and sticky hairs; leaves alternate, large, oval, lanceolate, sessile, deeply sinuous at the edges, soft, velvety, and sticky. The flowers, almost sessile, facing one side, are yellow with purple veins; the calyx has 5 teeth, the corolla is funnel-shaped with 5 unequal and blunt divisions. The fruit is a capsule opening at its top by a sort of operculum. Henbane is very common on road margins and in uncultivated places; it flowers almost throughout the summer.

White henbane (Hyosc. albus) and yellow henbane (Hyosc. aureus) possess the same poisonous properties. The active principle is hyoscyamine, an alkaloid crystallized in needle-shaped crystals.

The symptoms and treatment are those of belladonna or atropine poisoning; death may occur due to cardiac paralysis or

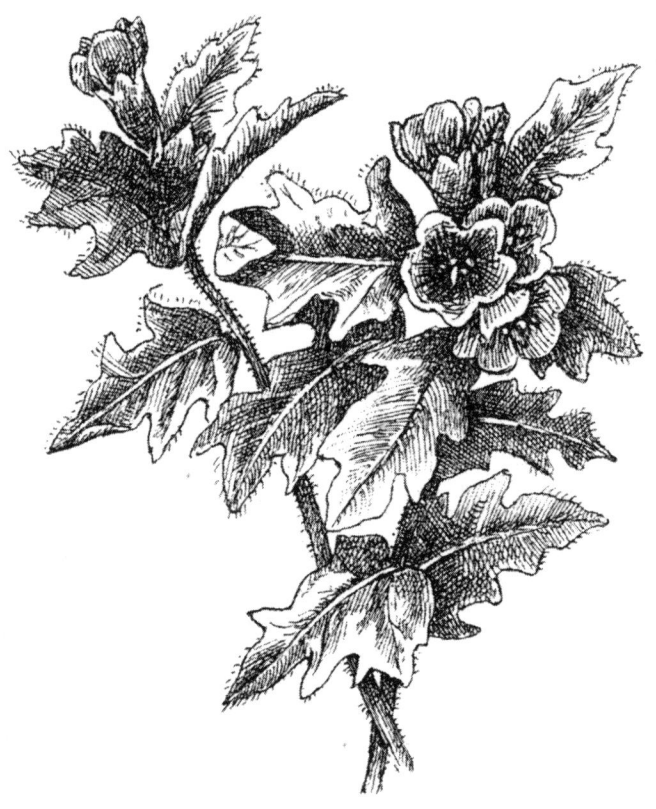

even apoplexy. *Wepfer* observed in one case transient madness. He recounts that one day by mistake he served the monks of the Rinhow convent henbane in a salad instead of chicory. After dinner, as was customary, the monks went to bed; but shortly afterward, they were struck by intoxication symptoms: general malaise, burning heat in the throat, dizziness. At midnight one monk was seized with delirium; his fellow brothers in the choir muttered disordered words, some saw ants, insects running on their books, others could not open their eyes. The next morning a tailor monk could not thread his needle, which he saw double and groped with his hand; no one died.

Datura (*Datura stramonium*, L.)

It is a large annual plant of the Solanaceae family. It has a herbaceous stem, somewhat hairy at its upper part, branching, ranging from 60 centimeters to 1.30 meters or more in height.

The leaves are large; velvety, oval, pointed; sinuous and angular, pedunculated. The flowers, white or violet, are very large; solitary, borne on a short peduncle; their calyx is tubular, elongated, marked by 5 protruding ridges that end up in as many uneven, sharp teeth; the corolla is funnel-shaped, with five very pronounced angles, ending up in five bent and pointed lobes. The fruit consists of an ovoid capsule, covered with spines, with four incomplete chambers communicating two by two and containing brownish, kidney-shaped seeds. This plant is native to India, but has acclimatized well in Europe. It is common in uncultivated places, near dwellings; it blooms in June and July; it also forms a vague ornament of gardens. All parts of the plant are poisonous. The active principle is daturine, which appears as white crystals soluble in water, alcohol, less soluble in ether.

Poisonings usually occur through ingestion by children of datura fruits; *Taylor* cites several cases of death, one of a two-year-old child who had swallowed about a hundred stramonium seeds,

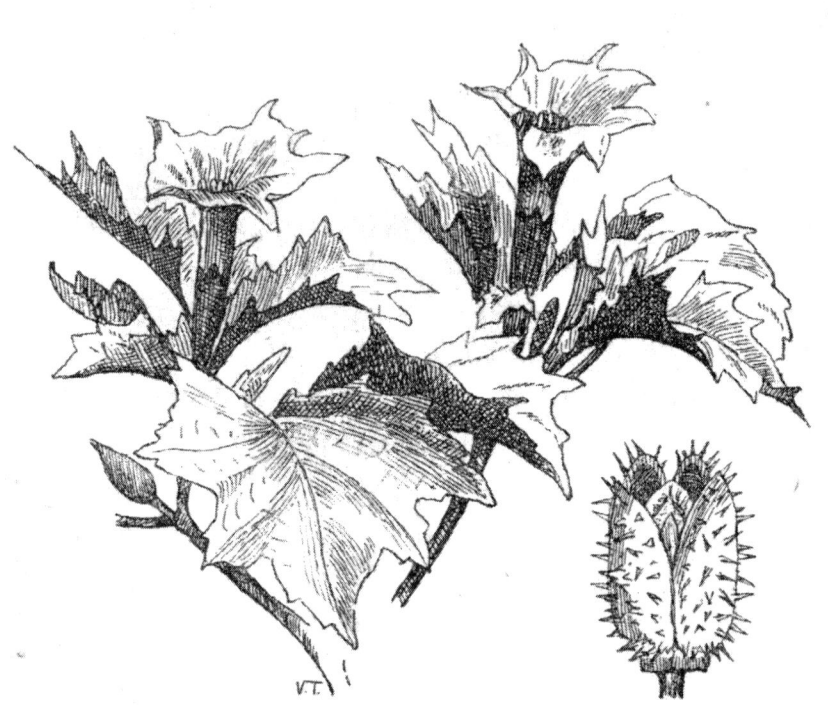

and one of a woman who knowingly administered to her mother a decoction of powdered datura seeds, about 125 in number; death followed in 7 hours. However, it is rare for the incidents produced by stramonium to be fatal; out of 51 cases collected by *Giraud* at the Bombay hospital, only one was lethal, and only four presented alarming symptoms.

The symptoms are similar to those of belladonna and henbane poisoning; only a more pronounced sexual excitement is observed.

The treatment is identical to that for belladonna intoxication.

II - Poisons with predominantly spinal action

Nux vomica (Strychnos nux vomica)

In India, particularly in Ceylon, Malabar, and on the Coromandel Coast, grows the tree whose seeds are commercially known as nux vomica.

The trunk of this Loganiaceae is of moderate height and thickness; the branches are opposite, glabrous, greenish, with opposite leaves on short petioles, smooth and oval. The flowers are small, white, forming terminal corymbs. The fruits are ovoid, almost as large as an orange, with a crustaceous and very fragile covering; the seeds, which appear scattered in a watery pulp, are orbicular, flattened, umbilicated on one of their faces, 14-18 millimeters wide with a thickness of 7-9 millimeters, grayish in color, with a bitter and disgusting taste.

The main toxic principles contained in these seeds are two alkaloids: strychnine and brucine. Strychnine ($C^{21}H^{22}N^2O^2$) appears as a white substance, crystallized in anhydrous quadrilateral prisms, poorly soluble in water, very soluble in alcohol and chloroform, almost insoluble in ether, with an extremely bitter taste. Brucine ($C^{25}H^{26}N^2O^4+4H^2O$) crystallizes in 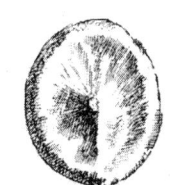 transparent and colorless prisms, soluble in water and alcohol, insoluble in ether and in fatty oils, with a very bitter taste. It acts on the organism like strychnine, but its activity is ten or fifteen times lesser.

Strychnine is a very active poison, and its salts (sulfate, acetate, hydrochloride, nitrate) seem to have a toxic potency even greater than that of the pure alkaloid, or rather they act more promptly, because they are more soluble and consequently absorbed more quickly. This occurs quite slowly through the gastric mucosa, more quickly through the rectum. The effects are almost immediate when these salts are injected into the veins.In humans, a dose of 2 centigrams of hydrochloride or another soluble salt of strychnine, ingested at once, could be life-threatening, and a half-smaller dose by hypodermic injection would certainly be very dangerous (*Vulpian*).

According to *Tardieu*, fatal accidents can result from the ingestion, in a healthy person, of 3-5 centigrams of strychnine taken at once or in a very short span of time; *Taylor* estimates the lethal dose to be from 0.024 to 0.10. 15 centigrams of alcoholic extract of nux vomica were a lethal dose; the minimal lethal dose of nux vomica powder is one and a half grams, in a case reported by *Christison*.

Poisonings from strychnine or nux vomica are mostly accidental, due to a fatal error in the administration of therapeutic doses, or because strychnine is taken for some other medicinal substance (in a case cited by *Danvin* it had been given instead of santonin).

A notable case of accidental poisoning for its uniqueness is that which happened to a Russian pharmacist. He had put in his pocket two capsules containing a few centigrams of strychnine each, intended for poisoning dogs, and in the same pocket, he had placed six cigarettes, which he smoked in the morning. At noon, feeling an inexplicable malaise, he searched for the capsules and realized that one had opened and the content had spilled onto the cigarettes. The doctors, immediately called, noted the symptoms of strychnine intoxication, symptoms that worsened to opisthotonos and cyanosis. Only three days later did these symptoms dissipate, and the patient was able to get up and walk.

Criminal poisonings are highly challenging due to the extremely bitter taste of these substances, even in minimal doses.

Nux vomica and its alkaloids act by violently stimulating the nerve centers, especially those located in the spinal cord; an increase in blood pressure and temperature is also noted; the psychic centers usually remain unharmed, at least until serious circulatory disturbances and symptoms of asphyxiation occur.

Symptoms and course of poisoning. - The course of strychnine poisoning includes three phases: a prodromal period, a convulsive period, and a period of exhaustion..

10-20 minutes after ingestion, symptoms begin with a sense of distress and increasing restlessness, soon followed by more severe phenomena. After some spasms and tonic contractions, the body arches in opisthotonos, then trismus occurs, violent convulsions followed by limb rigidity, dyspnea; the face, initially pale, becomes swollen and cyanotic, speech interrupted; death seems imminent, but shortly after the contractions cease, the muscles relax; a brief period of calm ensues. A new and more violent attack follows the first; the convulsions and opisthotonos reach their maximum intensity, voice emission is impossible, heartbeats are weak and irregular, the eyes are fixed and protruding, the pupils dilated, the skin becomes cyanotic, the patient is usually unconscious. The face is contracted in a "sardonic smile". This second attack is followed by a period of remission; sensitivity and consciousness return, circulation and respiration are restored, rarely perfect freedom of movement. Shortly, more frequent and intense attacks occur; sensitivity is so heightened that the slightest noise, minimal contact, merely speaking loudly in the patient's room or their efforts to eat or drink are enough to provoke a violent attack. Finally, a new attack, ending rapidly with death by asphyxia or exhaustion paralysis of the nervous system, concludes this dreadful scene.

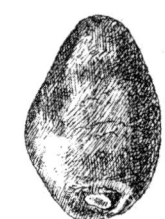

The attacks usually last no more than 3-4 minutes and the intervals are also very brief, so that death can occur within 1-2 hours after ingestion of the poison.

In more favorable cases, the attacks gradually diminish in intensity and dissipate within a few hours, leaving only severe physical and moral exhaustion; sometimes muscular rigidity persists in a limb or another part of the body.

Anatomical lesions. - The brain, spinal cord, meninges, lungs, pleura, and other internal organs show intense congestion that can progress to apoplexy. A cadaveric rigidity stronger than normal is also noted, which, according to Taylor, can last up to 8 days.

Treatment. - Emetics, gastric lavage, purgatives (castor oil). Tincture of iodine, tannin or tannic preparations to neutralize the poison.

For the convulsions, narcotics such as chloral, paraldehyde, chloroform, potassium bromide, morphine can be used; curare may also be tried. Methylal is also recommended as an antidote for strychnine. Artificial respiration has saved patients from asphyxiation in certain cases.

It is generally recognized that once symptoms of poisoning appear, they rapidly progress either towards recovery or death, and that the poison is so promptly eliminated that if the patient survives 2 hours, the likelihood of recovery is great, and practically certain after 4 or 5 hours..

Besides nux vomica, strychnine is found in other plants of the Strychnos genus; especially in the bark of false angostura and in St. Ignatius's bean.

The *bark of false angostura* comes from India in thick, compact, heavy plates with a grayish-red epidermis and gray internal matter; its powder is yellowish-white.

St. Ignatius's bean is the seed of a giant strychnine plant (Ignatia amara, L.). These seeds are irregularly ovoid and angular, about 2-3 centimeters long, with a pale brown striped surface, horny, hard, and greenish pulp, with an excessively bitter taste. They are found, 15-25 in number, scattered in the pulp of a fruit as large as an ordinary pear, ovoid, with a dry and fragile outer covering.

Semen contra

There are two main varieties of Artemisia that provide the drug known in trade as "semen contra" or "holy seed," which are Artemisia Contra and Artemisia Judaica. The former is indigenous to Persia and Asia Minor, while the latter grows especially in Arabia and ancient Judea. They are shrubs measuring 30-60 centimeters tall, with a branched, hairy stem of an ash-gray color, small oval leaves with several lobes, yellowish small pedunculate flowers forming a type of very long panicle. The fruits are ovoid, elongated, somewhat striated.

"Semen contra" is a mixture of flowers, fruits, and crushed twigs; it has a pleasant smell and aromatic taste, somewhat similar to that of anise. From it, a very active substance is extracted: santonin ($C^{15}H^{18}O^3$), crystallized in elongated quadrilateral, brilliant, colorless, odorless, tasteless tables. When treated with caustic potash in an alcoholic solution, it turns a scarlet red liquid that gradually discolors. It is insoluble in water, soluble in alcohol and ether, and its solution is very bitter; with lime, barite, and lead oxide it forms crystallizable salts. *Heldt* demonstrated that it combines with bases and can be considered as an anhydride of santoninic acid. Five centigrams of santonin are enough to cause poisoning in frail and anemic children; 25-30 centigrams constitute a lethal dose for children. 50 centigrams or 1 gram cause severe poisoning in an adult.

Symptoms of poisoning. - Mainly consist of visual disturbances: photophobia, xanthopsia (objects appear tinted yellow), scintillating scotomas, mydriasis, amblyopia, and transient amaurosis. *De Martiny* observed in the same individual, after 3 decigrams, yellow vision; after 6 decigrams, red vision, and after half an hour, yellow vision again; in another individual, he noted green vision, and in another, blue vision.

Schultze believes that this phenomenon depends on the yellow coloring of the ocular media or retina; *Hüfner* and *Helmholtz* attribute it to a direct action of santonin on the retinal elements that perceive violet, whose sensitivity first increases and then decreases. The gastroenteric phenomena are nausea, sometimes vomiting, meteorism, colic, diarrhea. In addition, there are circulatory and respiratory disturbances: slowing of the pulse with a lowering of temperature, dyspnea, difficult and stertorous breathing, and, besides visual disturbances, other nervous symptoms: hallucinations of hearing and smell, drunkenness, headache, prostration, drowsiness, and in severe cases, loss of consciousness, general body tremors, trismus, tonic and clonic convulsions resembling epileptic or tetanic fits. Sometimes cutaneous rashes (urticaria) and profuse sweating appear. The urine stains the linen yellow; their quantity is often increased. Death occurs after 15-48 hours in deep coma and more often amidst generalized convulsions.

Bertoni and *Raimondi*, in an adult man following the ingestion of 25 grams of santonin, noted: vomiting, dizziness, exceedingly severe prostration, cyanosis of the face, dyspnea, fainting spells, repeated epileptiform fits; however, recovery occurred.

Treatment. - Emetics, purgatives. Stimulants (coffee, ether, etc.). Oxygen inhalations, artificial respiration. Against convulsions: chloral, chloroform inhalations, etc.

Aniline (C⁶H⁵NH²)

Aniline is found among the products of dry distillation of fossil carbon and indigo; it was first prepared with indigo, which in Portuguese is called "anil." It is a colorless, oily liquid, slightly soluble in water, and very soluble in alcohol and ether. Treated with oxidizing agents, it yields a base, rosaniline, which is colorless in its free state, but when combined with acids and alcoholic radicals, gives rise to a series of bright and vivid colors. Aniline dyes are mostly harmless, provided they do not contain free aniline or other toxic substances (phenic acid, arsenic, lead, mercury).

Aniline acts on the nervous centers by violently stimulating them, similar to strychnine, and on the peripheral nerves by paralyzing them, like curare (*Filenhe*); it also has a very marked poisonous action on blood cells..

Acute poisoning. - Acute poisoning due to ingestion of toxic doses of aniline and aniline dyes presents the same symptoms as poisoning by oil of mirbane and requires the same treatment.

Inhaled aniline vapors produce headaches, dizziness, sometimes nausea and vomiting, numbness, cerebral congestion. The individual falls to the ground, makes some automatic movements, and breathes with difficulty. After about an hour, they come out of this crisis with an overwhelming drowsiness; in other cases, tetanic rigidity of the neck and epileptiform seizures alternating with delirium and general tremor occur (*Bergeron*). Breathing is irregular, convulsive, the skin is anesthetic, and the tongue, lips, and limbs are cyanotic; also observed are mydriasis, weak, slow, irregular heart beats. These symptoms usually vanish after an hour or more, leaving extreme exhaustion and intense headache.

Chronic poisoning. - This is most commonly observed in workers at aniline factories and is characterized by analgesia and anesthesia of the arms, sexual weakness and general exhaustion, cyanosis of the lips, and in more severe cases by visual disturbances, dysuria and strangury, dizziness, violent headache, cyanosis, nausea, and anorexia, uncertain and staggering gait, and sometimes even by loss of consciousness, cutaneous anesthesia, miosis, vomiting.

Treatment. - Prevention concerns good ventilation of laboratories. It will be good for workers to keep a small cloth or sponge soaked in an alkaline solution in front of their mouth.

Once the symptoms of intoxication have manifested, the patient should leave the laboratory for a few days, and in the meantime use alcohol and inhale ammonia vapors (*Dujardin-Beaumetz*).

Blister Beetles (*Lytta vesicatoria*).

These insects, commonly known as "Spanish flies" or "blister beetles," belong to the order Coleoptera. They measure 15-20 millimeters in length, with black, thread-like antennae, and flexible, elongated elytra that exhibit a golden green hue with metallic reflections.

They emit a characteristic, penetrating, and unpleasant odor; their taste is exceedingly bitter.

They appear in summer and are mainly found on ash and lilac trees, feeding on the leaves. To collect them, the trees on which they rest are shaken early in the morning, before sunrise, and the beetles fall onto sheets laid out on the ground; they are then killed by exposing them to the vapors of boiling vinegar and dried with the heat of a stove.

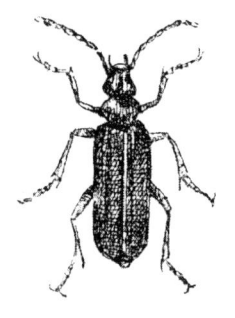

The active principle extracted from these beetles is cantharidin ($C^{10}H^{12}O^4$) which crystallizes in prisms or rhomboidal plates. It is a white substance, highly soluble in alcohol and ether, but insoluble in water.

Some animals, such as hedgehogs and chickens, are insensitive to the effects of cantharidin, even when injected subcutaneously; the flesh of chickens that have consumed blister beetles for an extended period becomes poisonous.

Blister beetle poisoning typically occurs through the ingestion of the powder or the alcoholic or ethereal tincture of blister beetles; however, it can sometimes result from the mere application of vesicants.

Small doses of blister beetles can be ingested over a long period without causing severe symptoms. *Frestel* reported the case of six students who, dining together, seasoned their food with blister beetle powder instead of pepper, and did not realize the mistake until several months later. During this time, they suffered only from back and kidney pains; only one was affected by simple urethritis, none by priapism.

According to *Tardieu,* the toxic dose of blister beetle powder is 40-50 centigrams for an adult, with the lethal dose being 1-2 grams; the toxic dose of the tincture of blister beetles is 24-30 grams, and that of cantharidin is 5 centigrams.

Symptoms and course of poisoning include intense burning in the mouth, throat, and stomach, with signs of severe gastroenteritis: sometimes bloody vomiting, excruciating colic pains, bloody diarrhea with extremely painful tenesmus.

Additionally observed are ptyalism, swelling of the salivary glands and tonsils, headache, prostration, fever of varying degrees, rapid and feeble pulse, and dyspnea. Severe irritation of the sexual organs presents as priapism or nymphomania, erotic or furious delirium; sometimes tetanic convulsions are observed. Urination is suppressed or minimal, containing blood and albumin, and extremely painful. In women, metrorrhagia and miscarriages in pregnant individuals are common.

In some cases, death occurs within one or two days, amidst convulsions or in profound coma.

Anatomical lesions include blisters and ecchymoses or ulcerations frequently observed on the mucous membrane of the gastrointestinal tract, especially in the stomach. The kidneys are intensely injected, inflamed, edematous, sometimes the site of hemorrhages; intense inflammation is also found in the urinary bladder and the external genital organs, which may appear gangrenous.

Treatment involves avoiding fatty substances that dissolve cantharidin; administer albumin water and mucilaginous drinks in abundance, camphor, opiates. Purgatives (calomel). Otherwise, symptomatic treatment (warm baths, etc.)..

III - Stimulant of the Brain and Spinal Cord

Camphor ($C^{10}H^{16}O$)

The Laurus camphora is a large tree that grows in the mountainous regions of the eastern parts of India, particularly in Japan. Camphor is a volatile oil with a unique concrete nature; it is abundantly found in all parts of this tree. To extract it, branches and roots, cut into pieces, are placed inside large iron kettles filled with water and topped with earthen lids. When heated moderately, camphor sublimates onto the rice straw lining the inside of the lid. In this state, it is impure, consisting of irregular gray masses; in Europe, it is purified and marketed.

Camphor acts by powerfully stimulating the central nervous system and the circulatory apparatus, resulting in increased blood pressure and the strength of heart contractions.

Symptoms of poisoning include excitement lasting only a few hours following the ingestion of small doses of camphor; for higher doses (several grams), there is initially a period of psychic exaltation and convulsions with dyspnea, temperature reduction, followed by anesthesia, paralysis of the rectum and bladder, collapse, death.

Mary Finley witnessed the death of a child who ingested 1 gram of camphor, and a woman who took 11 grams to induce abortion; she achieved her goal, however, she died in convulsions.

Orfila reports the observation of a healthy and robust twenty-year-old man, who, finding himself in a druggist's shop while camphor was being broken up to be put into bottles, began to chew on pieces, ingesting several grams. Soon after feeling tormented by a violent headache, without suspecting the cause, he left the store in a state of great exhilaration and upon meeting a friend, proposed a game of whist. After arriving home, his speech and actions became strange and singularly bizarre. Suddenly, he left his game, entered his room, and shortly emerged completely naked, dancing and attempting to jump out the window. Following the administration of opium, he vomited and became drowsy; he fully recovered within a few days.

Treatment includes emetics, gastric lavage. For convulsions: chloral hydrate, paraldehyde, inhalations of ether or chloroform. For collapse: stimulants (ether, coffee, etc.), cutaneous revulsives.

Turpentine Essence ($C^{10}H^{16}$)
(*Turpentine Oil*)

It is a clear liquid with a penetrating and aromatic odor, commonly used in the arts and industries, where it is better known as white spirit.

Prolonged exposure to an atmosphere containing turpentine vapors can be dangerous; *Méniere* reports that three workers, having descended into a well where 50 liters of turpentine had been spilled, became comatose and were barely saved; *Marchal de Calvi* observed the death of an individual who had slept in a room whose furniture had been freshly varnished with turpentine.

The lethal dose of turpentine essence is highly variable; *Mial* saw a child die within 15 hours after ingesting 15 grams of the essence; *Thomsen* noted a death case in an adult who had drunk 150 grams; however, there are also cases of recovery even after large doses (a glass).

Symptoms of poisoning include a sense of internal heat and dryness in the mouth and throat, ptyalism, nausea, vomiting with the smell of the essence, severe colic, meteorism, and diarrhea; headache, dyspnea, a feeble pulse, and cooling of the extremities are also observed; collapse, death in the deepest coma due to respiratory arrest.

At other times, a kind of drunkenness is observed with staggering gait, delirium, spasms, and convulsions, dysuria, strangury; painful erections. In the urine, albumin and fibrinous cylinders can be found; various exanthemas (erythema; papules, vesicles) may appear on the skin..

Anatomical lesions include severe hyperemia of the meninges and kidneys, hemorrhagic infarcts in the lungs and liver. The stomach and intestines appear edematous, with desquamated epithelium, ecchymosis, and small apoplectic foci; the blood is dark; droplets of turpentine essence can be found in the blood clots of the heart and vessels.

Treatment includes emetics, gastric lavage. Mucilaginous and emollient drinks. Stimulants (coffee, ether, etc.). Cutaneous revulsives, oxygen inhalations, artificial respiration.

Petroleum.

Petroleum is a mixture of various hydrocarbons: propane, butane; normal pentane, dimethylmethane, and paraffin.

The physiological action of petroleum has been little studied; from what can be gathered from the few clinical observations, it behaves almost analogously to turpentine oil (*Nothnagel*).

Inhaled, petroleum vapors can cause asphyxiation with pupillary miosis, cyanosis, lowering of temperature, and slowing of pulse and respiration. Ingested in rather large doses (an ordinary glass), this liquid produces palpitations, dizziness, shortness of breath, a small pulse (*Clemens*).

For larger doses, dyspnea, a weak and slow pulse, severe general malaise with a faint voice or constriction in the throat, ptyalism, constipation, anuria or oliguria with albuminous urine, miosis, and insensitivity of the pupils to light, prostration, lowering of temperature, collapse, loss of consciousness are noted. In other cases, violent tonic or clonic convulsions, extreme excitement, jaundice are observed.

However, sometimes even very large doses cause only mild disturbances; a worker, after drinking 200 grams of petroleum, experienced only some nausea and slight diarrhea.

In cases of poisoning, magnesium, albumin water, emetics, and purgatives are given. The collapse is fought with stimulants (coffee, alcohol, ether, etc.) and cutaneous revulsives (mustard plasters). Ice on the head.

PARALYZING POISONS

I - Poisons with cerebral action.

Sleepy Poppy (*Papaver somniferum*, L.)

The sleepy poppy is an annual plant, native to Persia and the Orient, but it thrives well in our climates too, and is cultivated for the ornamentation of gardens. The root is white, fusiform; the stem is straight, 50-80 centimeters high, glabrous; the leaves are sessile, elongated, acute, incised and toothed on the margins. The flowers are solitary, terminal; the calyx consists of 2 oval, concave, glabrous sepals; the corolla has 4 large white petals, or purplish with a brown spot at the base, blooming in June. The capsule, or poppy head, is ovoid, the size of a hen's egg, straw-yellow when dry, odorless, with a bitterish taste; it contains a large quantity of tiny white seeds, which, when pressed, yield poppy oil, used for the same purposes as olive oil.

This capsule develops and ripens shortly after the flower falls; at the appropriate time, which cultivators know wonderfully well, a worker enters the poppy field early in the morning, and,

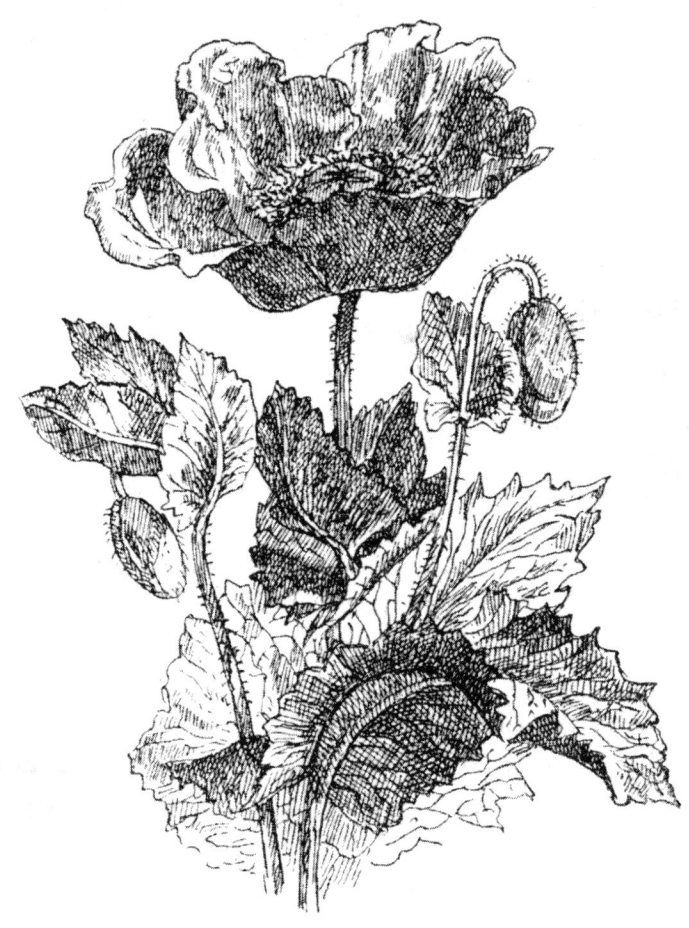

face turned towards the east, hand armed with an instrument with several parallel blades, similar in everything to a scarifier, incises the capsules in a spiral line directed from top to bottom. Thus, numerous laticiferous vessels are opened, and a white, milky juice drains and collects in a single drop at the lower part of the incision. This drop condenses, by evaporation, into a solid and dark tear, which constitutes the opium of the purest and most prized quality. A lower quality is prepared by grinding the capsules, stems, and leaves and evaporating the obtained liquid with pressure. The poppies that provide the opium of commerce are cultivated in India, Egypt, China, Persia, and Asia Minor.

Opium is usually put on the market in loaves of variable weight, wrapped in poppy, tobacco, or rumex leaves. It is a brown substance, with a penetrating and unpleasant odor, nauseating and bitter taste, soluble in water; it softens with heat and ignites if thrown on burning coals. The best quality is that of Smyrna, which contains 13-14% morphine, while that of Constantinople contains 10-12%, and that of Egypt only 2-3%.

Opium was in the past and still is today the object of careful studies and numerous researches; the alkaloids found so far, about forty, would be: morphine, apomorphine, codeine, narcotine, narceine, thebaine, papaverine, hydrocotarnine, etc. We will briefly mention the most important ones.

Morphine ($C^{17}H^{19}NO^3+H^2O$) crystallizes in rhomboidal prisms, translucent, colorless, shiny. It is odorless, with an extremely bitter taste, soluble in water and alcohol, almost insoluble in ether, chloroform, fatty and volatile oils. It forms crystallizable compounds with acids, generally soluble, the main ones being acetate, hydrochloride, and sulfate.

Apomorphine ($C^{17}H^{17}NO^2$) is initially colorless, but quickly oxidizes in contact with air, taking on a green tint. It is partly soluble in water, alcohol, ether, chloroform. It forms crystallizable salts with acids.

Codeine ($C^{18}H^{21}NO^3+H^2O$) crystallizes in large rhomboidal prisms; it is odorless, bitter, soluble in water, very soluble in alcohol and chloroform, absolutely insoluble in gasoline. It forms crystallizable salts with acids.

Narcotine ($C^{22}H^{23}NO^7$) crystallizes in shiny prisms, odorless, tasteless. It is insoluble in cold water, soluble in alcohol, ether, fixed and essential oils, dilute acids.

Narceine ($C^{23}H^{29}NO^9+H^2O$) crystallizes in colorless prismatic needles, silky, gathered in light masses, odorless, bitter, soluble in

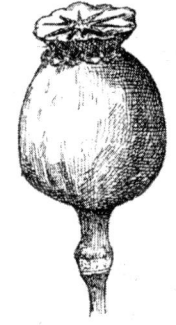

water and alcohol. Treated with a 2% iodine solution, it gives a beautiful characteristic blue color.

Thebaine, or paramorphine ($C^{19}H^{21}NO^3$) crystallizes in quadrangular flakes, with an acrid and astringent taste rather than bitter. It is very slightly soluble in cold water, soluble in alcohol, chloroform, gasoline, little in ether. Sulfuric acid stains it red.

Papaverine ($C^{21}H^{21}NO^4$) crystallizes in colorless prisms, insoluble in water, soluble in alcohol and ether. It forms crystallizable salts with acids.

Of these components, three have hypnotic virtues: morphine, narceine, codeine. Regarding their toxicity, in decreasing order, the following should be placed: thebaine, codeine, papaverine, narcotine, and morphine; and, in terms of their convulsant power, thebaine, papaverine, narcotine, codeine, and morphine.

Opium and morphine act by paralyzing the cerebral centers, subsequently paralyzing the respiratory center (which can be regarded as the principal, if not sole, cause of death); they also cause an increase in the reflex excitability of the spinal cord.

Acute poisoning by opium and its components

(*Thebaism and acute morphinism*) - Of all poisonings, those by opium or opiates are the most frequent, due to the numerous pharmaceutical preparations based on this narcotic, and their exceedingly frequent use, making accidental poisonings or those for suicidal purposes easy; as for criminal poisonings, they are much rarer.

Among the therapeutic preparations we note: simple opium tincture, Sydenham's and Rousseau's laudanum, opium extracts and syrups, Dower's powder, various analgesic ointments, etc., all medicines endowed with considerable activity.

Absorption is prompt and easy not only through the gastroenteric mucosa but also through the skin, even if intact. *Tardieu* observed a fatal poisoning through the application on the abdomen of a poultice that had been smeared with 30 grams of laudanum; *Christison* cites the case of a 32-year-old soldier who died within a few hours from complete narcotism following the application, during a facial erysipelas, of a compress soaked with an equal amount of laudanum on the inflamed skin; *Blache* noted alarming symptoms in two young women following laudanum plasters placed on the temples. Through skin deprived of the epidermis and the subcutaneous cellular tissue, the poison is absorbed even more readily, as is the case through the mucosa of the respiratory pathways; *Taylor* reports the case of a lethal poisoning due to the inhalation of a snuff powder into which morphine had been accidentally introduced.

It is noteworthy that healthy and robust individuals are generally more sensitive to opium and opiates than frail and sickly ones; an injection of 15 gr of morphine caused fatal poisoning in a very robust adult. Children show a great intolerance for these medications; 1 milligram of opium can kill a newborn, 2-3 milligrams a child not yet five years old; *Everest, Christison* reported fatal cases in newborns for only two drops of opium tincture or Sydenham's laudanum; 20 centigrams of Dower's powder were enough to kill a five-and-a-half-year-old child; *Tardieu* saw in one case a few spoonfuls of poppy decoction, administered by enema to a 6-week-old child, cause fatal accidents. Children can also be poisoned when the woman who nurses them has undergone treatment with opiates. Evans administered for about 3 days approximately 15 grams of "Liquor opii sedativus" to a woman in labor, suffering from strong uterine pain. On the fourth day, this woman breastfed a robust child, who nursed twice in 3 hours. Five hours later, Evans was called and found the child almost asleep, with slow and calm breathing, moist skin, and pupil myosis. Despite the administration of strong coffee, the child died 10 hours later. It follows that, after the use of opiates, breastfeeding should not be permitted.

Women are also very sensitive, so much so that 2-5 centigrams of morphine, by hypodermic injection, can sometimes cause serious poisoning.

Symptoms and course of poisoning. - The manifestation of symptoms is generally very rapid, half an hour or an hour after ingestion (in children even after a few minutes); first, there is severe fatigue with headache and heaviness of the head, dizziness, sensory hallucinations, delirium. A warm heat is spread throughout the body, the skin is the site of intense itching, sometimes of a vesicular or papular eruption; nausea ensues followed sometimes by vomiting, a sense of dryness in the mouth and throat; urine is scant or suppressed.

To this first period of excitement soon follows a state of severe stupor with loss of consciousness; gradual slowing of the pulse and breathing and lowering of temperature, mydriasis, and insensitivity of the pupils to light, relaxation of the muscles, coma, and sometimes (especially in children) convulsions and death due to cardiac and respiratory paralysis in a few hours (5-15) or in a few days.

In fortunately not rare cases, instead, a progressive improvement of symptoms is observed; the secretions are restored, and after severe weakness that lasts several days, there is a slow recovery.

In other cases, poisoning manifests immediately with profound coma followed by general paralysis and death within a few hours (1-2), sometimes even in 40-50 minutes.

Anatomical lesions. - Congestion of the brain and lungs, ectasia of the urinary bladder. The gastric mucosa was sometimes found stained yellow with opium; the skin shows many widespread ecchymoses: the blood is black and fluid.

Treatment. - Firstly, the poison must be removed from the body using emetics (zinc sulfate, or better yet, tartar emetic for enema or intravenous injection) and with the stomach pump. This indication should be followed not only in recent cases but also in those occurring a few hours prior, because opiates are absorbed very slowly. Antidotes include tannin and tannic preparations, potassium iodide, black coffee. According to *Personali*, methylal (1-4 grams in a potion of 150 grams) would be a good antidote for morphine, and *Arpad Bokai* insists a lot on the antagonism of picrotoxin and morphine, and believes that this substance gives the best results in poisoning from opium and morphine.

The patient must be made to walk if possible; in any case, prevent them from sleeping. Stimulants are very useful (camphor, ether, etc.). In the threat of asphyxia, cold showers, oxygen inhalations, artificial respiration will be resorted to. *Johnston* and *Wood* highly recommend atropine and claim that even the most serious opium poisonings can be cured with it, as atropine stimulates the deeply depressed respiration, thereby introducing the necessary oxygen into the blood. Potassium permanganate, if administered while the morphine remains in the stomach, proves to be an effective antidote, being capable of completely decomposing equivalent doses of morphine.

Chronic poisoning (*chronic morphinism and thebaism*):

I - MORPHINOMANIA. - The very common and frequent use of hypodermic injections of morphine has been the cause of a new disease: morphinomania, not rarely encountered among the more educated and higher social classes, and especially in neuropathic and neurasthenic individuals.

Out of 100 morphine addicts, *Levinstein* counted 72 men and 28 women. Out of 100, the same author found 32 physicians, 8 physicians' wives, 1 physician's son, 2 deaconesses (charity nuns of the Reformed Church), 2 nurses, 1 midwife, 1 medical student, 6 pharmacists, 1 pharmacist's wife. This brief statistic would demonstrate how the ease of procuring the poison contributes to the spread of the disease.

According to *Charcot* the precursor phenomenon of morphinism is the actual suffering experienced by the patient when the injection is not administered or simply delayed.

Symptoms of morphinism rarely manifest before 5-7 months of abuse and consist mainly of loss of appetite, weight loss that can progressively lead to the most pronounced marasmus, sooty complexion of the face, visual disturbances (pupillary miosis, amblyopia and even amaurosis), palpitations, hoarseness, dyspnea. At a more advanced stage, new and more serious disorders occur: insomnia, nightmares, hallucinations, tremors of the hands and tongue, neuralgia, intellectual torpor, impotence; a febrile state that leads the wretched to the grave through slow exhaustion.

Attacks of delirium tremens in a cheerful form have sometimes been noted.

The cure consists in the immediate or gradual suppression of morphine, substituting other cerebral stimulants: coffee, alcohol, cocaine, etc.

According to *Mattison,* the cure must be based on three drugs: sodium bromide, codeine, and trional; he asserts that they form a combination of unsurpassable efficacy if properly used; and constitute a therapeutic method far superior to those hitherto admitted. Hot baths, active bodily exercise, hydrotherapy are also commendable. It is advisable to confine the patient in a health facility and to monitor them carefully after their recovery to prevent relapses.

II - OPIUM EATERS AND OPIUM SMOKERS. The habitual use

of opium is particularly widespread in Asia, especially in Turkey, India, and China, and constitutes a more prevalent and damaging social scourge in those regions than alcoholism may be for us. A man accustomed to eating opium is easily recognizable by his significant emaciation, the yellowish tint of his skin, the stooping posture, and the staggering gait. The opium eater consumes very little food; his moral and physical strength are depleted; he lives in a state of great apathy and complete degradation. The habit forces him to gradually increase the dosage of the poison, thereby consuming substantial quantities; but in advanced stages, the unfortunate suffer from excruciating neuralgia to which opium can no longer provide any relief; it is rare for them to reach the age of 40 years, with death occurring in the most severe state of wasting. Cases of opium eating were also noted in Europe, especially in England, and even more so, in America.

The practice of smoking opium is particularly common in China, and its effects are very similar to those produced by opium eating. Initially, there is a pleasurable excitement of the imagination; annoyances, boredom, and pains disappear, and the smoker is immersed in delightful lethargy. This is followed by a period of depression, with physical and intellectual weakness followed by heavy sleep that brings no refreshment. Smokers generally start with 5 pipes and over time can come to smoke up to 40-50 pipes a day; however, a habitual dose is only about 15-20 pipes. In older individuals, who have been smoking opium for many years, *Michaut* observed a paralysis similar to that caused by lead poisoning. As an important diagnostic difference, he noted the absence of alterations in sensitivity and the leaden line on the gums.

Indian Hemp (*Cannabis indica, L.*). or hashish

Hashish is very commonly used among Arabs, for whom it has become an imperative need just like opium for Orientals and alcohol for Northern peoples. This name refers to a plant whose active ingredient forms the main component of various intoxicating preparations widely used in Egypt, Syria, and almost all Eastern regions. This plant belongs to the family of Ulmaceae and is common in India and Southern Asia, where it grows wild; it resembles the European hemp very closely.

The most common preparation of hashish is a fatty extract, obtained by boiling the leaves and flowers of the plant in water with a certain amount of butter, and then evaporating the mixture down to a syrupy consistency, followed by filtering through a cloth. In this way, the butter becomes charged with the active principle and assumes a very distinct green color, but due to its unpleasant and nauseating taste, it is never used alone, but rather in the preparation of electuaries and pastes that are flavored with rose and jasmine essences, to mask the rather offensive odor of the pure extract.

The broader leaves of the plant are smoked like tobacco by the less affluent populations of India and are also used to prepare an intoxicating infusion. The active principle of Indian hemp is a resinous substance that was named cannabin.

In moderate doses, hashish induces a sort of pleasant intoxication, brightened by delightful dreams. Toxic doses cause violent headache, anxiety, nausea, vomiting, and a sense of severe malaise; however, the poison is ordinarily expelled with vomiting, and within a few hours, all disturbances have disappeared. Very strong doses lead to a heavy, distressing sleep, which leaves behind serious exhaustion.

The habitual use of this plant, as seen from numerous cases observed among Easterners, causes degeneration and can lead to imbecility and madness. Hashish eaters display a notable jaundiced tint to the skin and have a fixed and expressionless gaze and a stupid countenance.

II. Bulbar-acting Poisons.

Prussic Acid (CyN)

Hydrocyanic acid, also known as prussic acid, discovered by *Schéele* in 1780, is a colorless liquid with a penetrating odor similar to that of bitter almonds and is slightly soluble in water.

It is found in many plants, primarily in the leaves of cherry laurel and in bitter almonds of the Rosaceae family. The cherry laurel (*Prunus laurocerasus*, L.) is a shrub that can reach

6-7 meters in height, with a smooth, blackish trunk, persistent, always green, oval, elongated, pointed at the end, serrated on the margins, leaves that are shiny green on the upper side and paler beneath; when rubbed between fingers, they release the smell of bitter almonds; distilled with water they yield hydrocyanic acid, an essence ($C^{14}H^6O^2$)quite analogous to that of bitter almonds. 3-4 of these leaves can already produce symptoms of poisoning; the essence is extremely toxic; a single drop, placed on a dog's wound, is enough to kill it. The lethal dose of cherry laurel distilled water is 30 grams.

Bitter almonds are the seeds of the bitter variety of Amigdalus communis; they are very similar to sweet almonds, only somewhat smaller.

According to *Braithvaite,* bitter almond essence contains 4.1-6.3 percent hydrocyanic acid; that of cherry laurel contains a somewhat lesser amount.

Other plants also yield hydrocyanic acid, especially Ramnus frangula, the seeds of vetch and flax, the roots of Manihot esculenta, the fruits of Ximenia americana, the seeds of Lecythis ollaria and Chardinia xeranthemoides, the latex of Ipomoea carnea, and a mushroom, Amanita muscaria. In addition, varying amounts were found in the distilled waters of Arum maculatum, Ribes aureum, Aquilegia vulgaris, Poa aquatica, and especially in the products of distillation of Linum usitatissimum seed emulsion.

Poisoning by hydrocyanic acid is extremely rare due to the great difficulty in obtaining it; however, intoxication with preparations containing hydrocyanic acid, such as distilled waters and essences of bitter almonds (17 drops were enough

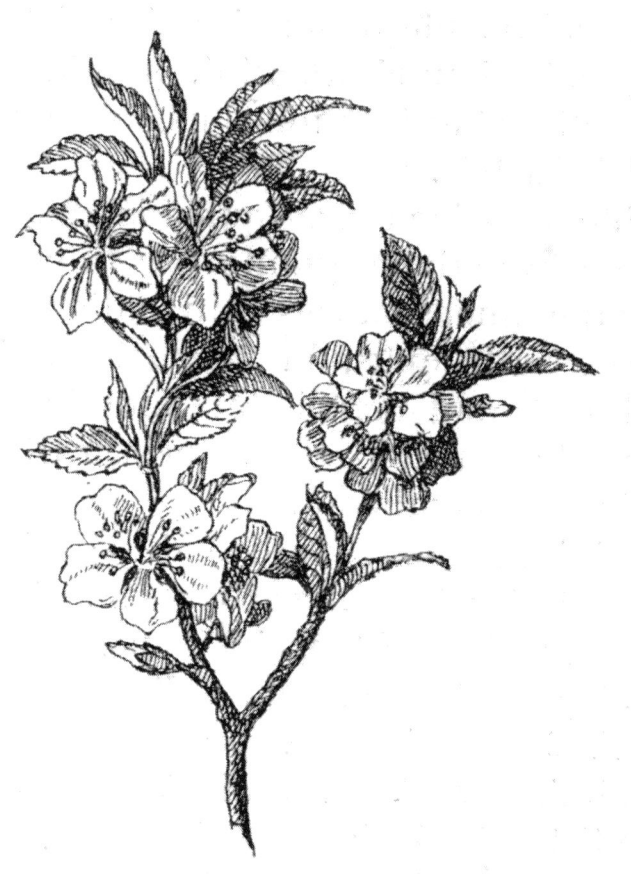

to kill a woman in half an hour) and of cherry laurel, with bitter almonds, with large amounts of cherry stone (30 grams produce 3-7 centigrams of hydrocyanic acid), with poorly flavored liquors with bitter almonds, with alkaline cyanides, especially with potassium cyanide, widely used in numerous arts and industries, are much more frequent.

Hydrocyanic acid acts almost instantaneously, whether by ingestion or by its application on accessible mucous membranes, the ocular conjunctiva, and the skin; its action is especially on the centers of the medulla oblongata, producing respiratory paralysis, slowing of the pulse, and convulsions.

The minimum lethal dose is 65 milligrams for an adult; however, cases of recovery have been observed after taking 8 and even 12 centigrams at once. Inhalation of its vapors (boils at 26° C!) produces very serious, often fatal phenomena; it is to one of these terrible accidents that the loss of *Scheele*, the famous chemist, is attributed. In the case observed by *Regnault*, it involved a student who was on the verge of death for having inhaled vapors that escaped from a vessel in which hydrocyanic acid had been prepared. This young man remained several hours in almost absolute coma; his face was cyanotic, the pupil was very dilated, breathing was labored and intermittent, the skin was cold, the pulse was almost imperceptible, and the muscles were agitated by clonic convulsions; for several days he suffered from a headache and severe prostration.

Symptoms and course of Poisoning. - Symptoms arise almost instantaneously; at most they may take a few minutes to appear. The poisoned individual staggers and falls like an inert mass, without uttering a word; their entire body is stiffened by tetanic convulsion, the face is swollen and cyanotic or pale, the eyes bulge from their sockets, the pupils are dilated, the mouth is covered with bloody foam. Subsequently, a few convulsions occur, then the body returns to its state of rigidity; the temperature drops rapidly, the pulse becomes imperceptible, and death occurs within a few minutes (2-15) or at most within three-quarters of an hour, after some alternations of convulsive paroxysms and coma, during which breathing is sometimes stertorous (*Tardieu*).

If the dose of the toxin is not lethal, besides the loss of consciousness, violent convulsive seizures are observed for 2-3 hours; the respiration is slow and spasmodic, the heartbeat weak, the skin cyanotic; trismus and muscle spasms are also noted. Subsequently, the patient gradually regains consciousness and intelligence, and sometimes vomiting occurs, a sign of good prognosis; a sense of general weakness persists for several days, followed by recovery.

Anatomical lesions. - Congestion of the brain, spinal cord, lungs, abdominal viscera, and the gastroenteric mucosa. The heart is filled with fluid, dense, bluish-black blood and sometimes with a cherry-red color. All parts of the corpse emit a strong odor of bitter almonds.

Treatment. - Emetics, gastric lavage. Cold affusions on the nape and along the spinal column. Faradization, artificial respiration. Stimulants (strong coffee infusion, ammonia, alcohol, ether, etc.).

As antidotes, atropine, hydrated iron oxide, chlorine water, and hypodermic injections with 5-10 percent solutions of sodium hyposulfite are recommended (*Lang*).

Potassium Cyanide (KCN)

This salt is white, odorless, with a caustic, alkaline, and bitter taste; it is highly soluble in water and less soluble in alcohol.

It is used in laboratories as a reducing agent, in gold and silver electroplating, and in photography. It is one of the most formidable poisons known; the symptoms are similar to those produced by prussic acid. Lethal doses vary from 5 to 10 centigrams.

Tardieu reports the case of a photographer who, wishing to remove the black stains on one of his hands left by silver nitrate, rubbed it with a large piece of potassium cyanide, and accidentally pushed a small fragment under the nail of a finger. Not paying immediate attention to it, he soon felt a sharp pain and became dizzy. To promptly rid himself of it, he had the misfortunate idea to use vinegar; the cyanide was quickly decomposed, releasing prussic acid. Dizziness reached maximum intensity, accompanied by chills, pallor of the face, profound prostration, inability to speak; then cooling of the extremities, diplopia; consciousness remained unaltered. This state lasted about ten hours, after which the symptoms disappeared following cold rubs on the spinal column, ammonia inhalations, and ingestion of a strong brew of black coffee.

The treatment is identical to that for cyanide poisoning. *Antral* claims to have cured forty people poisoned by potassium cyanide by administering cobalt nitrate to them, which combines with the cyanide to form an insoluble and harmless precipitate. *Kossa* considers potassium permanganate as the chemical antidote to potassium cyanide; it would prevent the paralysis of the respiratory centers.

Coca (*Eritroxilon coca*).

It is a shrub of the Linaceae family, ranging from half a meter to one and a half meters tall, very branched, with alternate, close, short-petiolated, oval or oval-lanceolate, membranous leaves, paler green on their lower surface. Only the leaves are used from the plant; they contain a crystallizable alkaloid, cocaine ($C^{17}H^{21}NO^4$). Coca is native to Peru, Bolivia, Brazil, and other regions of South America.

Acute cocaine poisonings are mostly accidental, due to injections of too high doses of the alkaloid for therapeutic purposes. *Dujardin-Beaumetz* and others have seen toxic accidents arise from hypodermic injections not exceeding 1-2 centigrams of cocaine. *Berger* observed a fatal case due to injection into the vaginal tunic of a spoonful of a 2% cocaine solution in a young man suffering from hydrocele. *Maltison* noted two lethal poisonings: one following injection into the urethra of one cubic centimeter of a 4% cocaine solution; the other due to injection into a facial nevus. *Delboxe* reported 4 cases followed by death for doses of 50-80 centigrams; *Abadie* a case of death in 5 hours following the injection of 4 centigrams into the lower eyelid; *Kolomnin* saw a woman die 3 hours after the administration of an enema containing 1.04 grams of cocaine.

Anemics, neuropaths, the elderly, children, the weak, heart and lung patients show a particular susceptibility to cocaine, and it appears that facial injections especially predispose to intoxication.

This alkaloid initially excites the spinal and medulla

oblongata; in a later period, it causes the cessation of respiratory movements due to paralysis of the medulla oblongata.

Symptoms of acute poisoning. - The symptoms of acute cocaineism appear very rapidly and consist of precordial anxiety, sometimes nausea and vomiting, restlessness, agitation, and often transient delirium, dyspnea, forceful cardiac beats, extremely frequent and threadlike pulse. There is also dizziness and vertigo, ringing in the ears, confusion of ideas, mydriasis, pallor of the skin. Sometimes, there is prostration, drowsiness, loss of consciousness.

Often these symptoms are joined by tonic and clonic spasms of the face and limbs, amid which death occurs due to syncope or tetanic arrest of the thorax and diaphragm. In more favorable cases, these accidents last a few hours or at most a few days, and complete recovery occurs. However, *Hallopeau* observed in one case persistent headache, insomnia, numbness and tingling of the limbs, and episodes of vertigo with fainting for four months.

Following the ingestion of 2 grams of cocaine in an adult, and 5 grams in a child, nothing but profound drowsiness lasting several days was observed, which dissipated without a trace.

Anatomical lesions. - They are not very characteristic; at autopsy, there is usually found intense congestion of the meninges, the lungs, and other internal organs.

Treatment. - The prophylaxis involves never injecting more than 2 centigrams of cocaine at a time, and administering the injection while the patient is in the supine position to avoid syncope due to cerebral anemia.

Once poisoning has manifested, the patient should be kept

in a horizontal position, and hypodermic injections of ether, caffeine, and morphine hydrochloride should be administered. Black coffee is recommended as a beverage. To modify arterial pressure and calm convulsions, inhalations of amyl nitrite, ethyl iodide, chloroform, and administration of chloral are resorted to.

In the event of asphyxiation, massage, oxygen inhalations, and artificial respiration may prove beneficial.

Chronic poisoning. - Prolonged use of cocaine, mostly in morphine addicts who have replaced morphine with cocaine, and habitual abuse of coca leaves can lead to intoxication characterized by circulatory disorders (tachycardia, frequency and irregularity of pulse), dyspnea, profuse sweating and diarrhea, syncope, delirium with illusions and hallucinations (the patient sees objects moving, changing in size and shape; hears buzzing, noises, voices; feels a tingling sensation, as if the skin were invaded by countless tiny animals. Seglas observed a patient who was not only certain of having such creatures under his skin but also believed he saw them under the skin of others approaching him and proposed their extraction with suitable instruments). Sometimes, a delirium of persecution is observed, driving the patient to desperate acts. In chronic cocaine use, there is also typically observed a loss of memory, weakness of will, insomnia, sexual impotence, combined with severe physical wasting, progressive and considerable emaciation.

The treatment consists of discontinuing the use of cocaine and combating the various morbid manifestations.

III - Spinal Poisons.

Phenic Acid (C⁶H⁶O).
(Phenol, carbonic acid).

Phenic acid, a product of the partial distillation of tar oil, is solid at room temperature and crystallizes into long, colorless needles with a smell similar to that of creosote and a pungent, burning taste; it greases paper like a fatty substance. It is highly deliquescent, soluble in water, and extremely soluble in alcohol, ether, chloroform, glycerin, and in fixed and volatile oils.

Phenic acid is readily absorbed by the mucous membrane of the digestive tract, by cellular tissue, from the surface of sores and wounds, and even through intact skin. Rubbing onto the skin and dressings made with a phenic acid solution could cause fatal intoxication, with the same symptoms observed following ingestion of the poison. *Küller*, among 5 cases of poisoning from phenic acid dressings, saw 4 end in death. 1-2 grams are enough to produce serious, sometimes fatal, poisoning; a smaller dose may suffice for women and children; alcoholics may acquire a special idiosyncrasy, whereby they would tolerate phenic acid better than others.

At high doses, this acid leads to paralysis of the spinal cord; the motor and sensory nerves and the muscles remain intact (*Summer Stone*).

Symptoms of poisoning. - These consist mainly of headache, dizziness, stupor, ringing in the ears with hypoacusia, a tingling sensation, exhaustion, and severe weakness. There is also profuse sweating, slow pulse, lowered temperature, and gastroenteric symptoms such as nausea, vomiting, enteralgia, diarrhea. The urine is olive green or gray-black; sometimes it contains hemoglobin and albumin (nephritis).

In severe cases, when the ingested dose is quite large, the patient complains of a burning sensation in the mouth, along the esophagus, and in the stomach; there is also a sort of intoxication quickly followed by loss of consciousness, sticky sweats, stupor, miosis, and insensitivity of the pupils to light, severe dyspnea, collapse, death by cardiac paralysis or asphyxia.

Rumbold observed in an individual who had drunk about a liter of crude phenic acid a rapid loss of consciousness, motor incapacity with muscle contractions without convulsions, coma and progressive respiratory distress, absence of vomiting, death by asphyxia.

Anatomical lesions. - The mucosa of the mouth, esophagus, and stomach often appear white, thickened, and corroded; the lungs were found congested with blood, the bronchi filled with tenacious, brownish-red mucus. In some cases, nephritis was observed.

Treatment. - Emetics, gastric lavage. The antidotes are lime water, calcium saccharate, sodium sulfate, albumin, milk. *Carleton* recommends the use of vinegar, claiming that even in internal poisoning by phenic acid, vinegar acts as a good antidote, and advising to drink vinegar diluted with water and then to perform gastric lavage. The collapse is fought with stimulants (coffee, ether, camphor, etc.). Oxygen inhalations, artificial respiration will prevent asphyxiation.

Creosote (C^7H^9O)

Creosote is an oily, transparent liquid with a very sharp smell reminiscent of smoked meat and a caustic taste; it is obtained through the distillation of wood tar.

The ingestion of concentrated creosote causes severe caustic burns in the stomach and intense gastroenteritis with dysuria and sometimes stranguary, urine in some cases is brownish and albuminous. Furthermore, serious nervous symptoms appear: headache, palpitations, dizziness, extreme distress, loss of consciousness, collapse, convulsions. Death is likely due to cardiac or diaphragmatic paralysis, or even, though very rarely, following acute peritonitis from perforation.

Anatomical lesions. - The organs give off a strong creosote smell; the brain and lungs are congested with black blood; blood clots fill the heart cavities; significant hyperemia is found in the kidneys and meninges.

Treatment. - The antidotes are albumin, and milk in large quantities. Emetics, gastric lavage. Symptomatic care.

Nitrobenzene ($C^6H^5NO^2$).
(Oil of mirbane, artificial bitter almond essence)

It is obtained by treating benzene with nitric acid. It is a clear liquid, yellowish in color, sweet in taste, with the smell of bitter almonds; almost insoluble in water, soluble in alcohol, ether, etc. This substance is widely used by perfumers and confectioners as a substitute for essential oil of bitter almonds.

Bergeron reported that nitrobenzene vapors can cause dizziness followed by coma; *Letheby* observed cases of death due to prolonged exposure in environments saturated with these harmful vapors.

Poisonings due to the ingestion of nitrobenzene are almost all accidental, caused by carelessness or inattention.

Symptoms of poisoning. - Burning heat in the mouth at the moment of ingestion, followed by a sense of numbness and tingling in the tongue and lips, heavy-headedness, anesthesia, weak pulse, bluish skin and soon notably cyanotic; the breath and urine of the patient emit a strong odor of bitter almonds.

In severe cases, in addition to loss of consciousness, there are still signs of trismus and convulsions..

Treatment. - Gastric lavage, emetics, stimulants, artificial respiration. *Strümpell* asserts having obtained excellent results with blood transfusion.

Phenacetin ($C_{10}H_{13}N_2O$)

It crystallizes in colorless needles; it is very slightly soluble in cold water, more soluble in alcohol and acetic acid.

Toxic doses of phenacetin produce phenomena of paralysis of the spinal cord and medulla oblongata, preceded by a short period of excitation (*Mahnert-Ubaldi*).

Hinsberg and *Krafft* noted that the ingestion of 3-5 grams of phenacetin induces, within three hours, an acceleration of the pulse and respiration with vomiting, cyanosis of the mucous membranes, and a comatose state; methemoglobin was found in the urine. *Fernandez de Harra* reported the case of a lady who was severely poisoned after ingesting two packets of 65 centigrams each of phenacetin, *Lindemann* observed intense cyanosis following the administration of 2 grams of the drug; *Von Yaksch* saw the same cyanosis appear after the administration of 10 and 20 centigrams in one individual with typhoid and another with pleurisy. In addition to cyanosis, various exanthemas were also observed, and *Muller* has drawn attention to a variety of diarrhea following the use of phenacetin; he also noted the increased severity of symptoms after the ingestion of 6-8 grams of this drug. Collapse phenomena were noted by *Krönig* in an eight-year-old child, who had ingested 50 centigrams of phenacetin. Other symptoms that are more frequently found in these poisonings include: heaviness of the head, dizziness, a sense of cooling, drowsiness, an extremely distressing sense of anguish, cold and abundant sweats, and convulsions.

Treatment. - Cardiac stimulants; inhalations of amyl nitrite.

IV - Paralyzers of the Brain and Spinal Cord.

Tobacco (*Nicotiana tabacum*, L.)

This solanaceous plant has an annual root, a straight, branched, cylindrical stem growing from 60 centimeters to 1.30 meters in height, hairy and sticky. The leaves are alternate, very large, oval, narrow at the base, sessile, hairy, 30 centimeters long, 8-10 centimeters wide. The flowers are large, pink, arranged in a sort of panicle at the end of the branches; the fruit is an ovoid capsule, opening into two valves.

Tobacco was found in Mexico by the Spaniards around 1520, near the city of Tabago. The Indians called it "petun" and used the leaves, which were previously prepared by burning and inhaling the smoke through long grass straws. However, only priests, and only on significant occasions, enjoyed this privilege; by intoxicating themselves with tobacco smoke, they would fall into a sort of ecstasy, during which they predicted the outcomes of the most important events. The Spaniards, having learned the use of tobacco from the Mexicans, brought it to Europe, particularly to Spain and Portugal, where its use spread everywhere, mainly through the work of the Jesuits. In 1560 or 1565 it was introduced into France during the reign of Charles IX; at this time, Nicot, the French ambassador to Lisbon, brought it as a gift to Catherine de' Medici. Hence the names "nicotiana" and "queen's herb," under which tobacco was first known. From France, it later spread to other northern regions of Europe; but only after overcoming a thousand obstacles did this practice become popular. In 1604, James I of England wrote a book against tobacco, and the Jesuits in response wrote in praise of the new plant. Pope Urban VIII, in 1624, threatened excommunication for those found sniffing tobacco in churches with a special bull. This prohibition extended to almost all the peoples of Europe, Persia, and Turkey, where the use of tobacco threatened nose amputation.

But later, governments, aware of the enormous financial benefits they could derive, allowed the use of tobacco, albeit heavily taxed.

Tobacco owes its toxicity to the presence of an alkaloid, nicotine, ($C^{10}H^{14}N^2$) a substance which, according to *Schroff*, is sixteen times more potent than coniine. This alkaloid, discovered by *Vauquelin*, is a transparent, colorless, oily, anhydrous liquid; it easily deteriorates in the air, becoming brown and thick; it is very soluble in water, with an acrid odor and a burning taste.

The lethal dose of nicotine, according to *Schroff*, is 2-16 centigrams; death occurs due to cerebral paralysis and of the inspiratory muscles.

Various types of tobacco contain nicotine in very different proportions: Alsatian and Havana tobaccos contain 2-3 percent; those from Virginia and the North 6-7 percent; and Eastern tobaccos contain very little.

The extremely toxic property of nicotine is well known and exploited in some regions of America for certain criminal practices. There, writes *Depierris* in his accurate and valuable monograph on tobacco, where life is quite easy, the rough trade of sailing has no allure, despite the generous wages attached to it, so often one must resort to fraud to provide ships with the necessary men. Real bands of thugs deal with the captains of merchant ships to give them on board, at the time of departure, the number of men they need. These human flesh traders then set about their abominable task; they eye in the streets the man who seems to suit them, surround him, seduce him with a thousand kindnesses, and end up leading him to some dive, where accomplices are already present. Once there, they ask the guest which drink he desires, and it is served in a glass that he sees taken from the counter. This glass is turned upside down, seems clean, nothing could suggest that the unfortunate will leave not only his reason but even his every sentiment. But what was done to give this glass such mysterious and terrible properties? Something very simple; a few puffs of tobacco smoke, blown into it before using, and the glass is poisoned! Its walls come to be covered with an invisible cloud of pure nicotine, which dissolves in the drink, whatever it may be, that the victim has asked for. The unlucky one drinks without tasting the flavor of tobacco, masked by the acridity of the drink and by the dense clouds of smoke with which the wretches are careful to surround him. As soon as he has swallowed this infernal potion, he is led out of the tavern; the narcotic exhilaration quickly takes hold, blurring his vision and numbing his senses. He is loaded onto a dinghy and hoisted aboard by a rope; he will not awaken from his nicotine stupor until he is at high sea, on the deck of a ship, with no recollection of how he arrived there.

The causes of tobacco poisoning are various; one of the most common and frequent is smoking. It is true that some of the nicotine is destroyed by combustion, but largely it accumulates at the bottom of the pipe bowl or at the back end of the cigar and can be absorbed. For this reason, pipes may be more harmful than cigars, as the combustion in them is slower and more incomplete. Besides nicotine, tobacco smoke contains many other poisonous volatile bases that are produced during combustion, such as pyridine, picoline, lutidine, and collidine; it also contains prussic acid, hydrogen sulfide, carbon monoxide, etc. There are, unfortunately, cases of fatal poisoning; one individual died after smoking 17 pipes consecutively; *Schroff* reported a case where just two pipes killed the smoker, and *Murray* noted a fatal poisoning of two brothers following 7-8 uninterrupted pipes. A vineyard worker, whose story was told by *Marrigues,* was luckier; he survived 25 consecutive pipes but suffered from it for over eighteen months. In the case observed by Camden, it was a two-year-old child who died within hours from sucking on an old pipe that belonged to his father.

Poisoning by ingestion of tobacco is quite rare; it sometimes occurs in the insane or in suicides. A few grams, taken in this way, can cause death; the lethal dose for snuff may be only 2 grams.

The most famous case of poisoning is that of the poet Santeuil, who died in excruciating pain after drinking a glass of Spanish wine into which snuff had been put. A madman swallowed 30-40 grams of tobacco; violent tetanic convulsions, profuse vomiting and diarrhea, thread-like pulse followed, then tetanic rigidity set in with death within 7 hours.

Enemas made with a decoction of tobacco leaves are very dangerous; fatal accidents have been caused by a dose of 8 grams in a fourteen-year-old child, of 30, 40, 60 grams in adults.

It is known that the nasal mucosa also has a considerable absorptive power; intoxication can result from the habit of snuffing tobacco; *Hutchinson* was able to note the frequency of amaurosis. It is recorded in the "Éphémérides des curieux de la nature" that an individual fell into a state of drowsiness and died of apoplexy after sniffing a large quantity of powdered tobacco.

Chewing tobacco, due to the more frequent ingestion of nicotine dissolved in saliva, is a more dangerous habit than smoking.

Applied to intact skin, and even more so to skin without its epidermis, tobacco can cause serious, often fatal, poisoning; unfortunately, there are numerous examples. *Namias*, in a note communicated to the Academy of Sciences of Paris, reported the case of a smuggler who had been applying tobacco leaves to his bare skin for months to evade taxes; the leaves, moistened by sweat, caused poisoning that healed with the use of alcohol and laudanum. *Hildenbrand* tells that the hussars of an entire squadron wrapped their bodies with tobacco leaves for smuggling purposes, and, although they were all heavy smokers, they were nevertheless poisoned. *Polk* noted the intoxication of a robust 37-year-old farmer following the application of tobacco leaves smeared with honey on his limbs to treat chronic rheumatism.

Poisonings were also noted after the application of tobacco juice on a chronic rash on the neck, after rubbings with this juice on bare skin parts, on ulcers or sores, after wrapping limbs with cloths soaked in a very hot concentrated infusion of tobacco.

Depierris finally cites the observation of three Chinese, two of whom died from having fallen asleep in a closed room where there were 60 kilograms of tobacco.

Symptoms of acute poisoning. - In mild cases, such as are ordinarily observed in novice smokers, the symptoms consist of headache, dizziness, a feeling of oppression in the epigastrium, nausea and vomiting, sialorrhea, pale skin covered in cold sweat.

In severe cases, usually due to ingestion or enemas of tobacco infusion, in addition to the previous symptoms, there is restlessness, delirium, pupillary dilation, dyspnea, very small, irregular, accelerated pulse, loss of consciousness, tetanic attacks, and in some cases death in profound collapse.

Treatment. - Emetics, purgative enemas, stomach pump. The antidotes are tannin and potassium iodide. For collapse, stimulants (coffee, ether injections, etc.) are used. Some recommend strychnine as an antagonist to nicotine.

Chronic Poisoning. - This is observed in those who habitually chew tobacco and in heavy smokers.

Although for this poison, as for many others, the majority of cases show a high tolerance on the part of the organism, this is never so perfect as to prevent, sooner or later, the fairly frequent occurrence of serious functional disorders. The main ones would be:

From the digestive tract: dyspepsia often associated with pharyngitis (granular pharyngitis) and constipation.

From the heart: palpitations, weakness of cardiac contractions, neurosis (angina pectoris)..

From the nervous system: apathy, intellectual torpor, sexual weakness or impotence, dizziness; insomnia, and in severe cases, delirium similar to that of alcoholics, mental derangement can be observed.

It is well-known that the majority of mad people are smokers; that tobacco is the true cause of madness in some is proven by the fact that the cessation of this bad habit is followed by the disappearance of all mental symptoms.

Disturbances in vision are not rare either: scintillating scotomas, amblyopia, amaurosis. The general nutrition of the organism is usually altered; there is an anemic state with weight loss, flaccidity, and muscular weakness.

Treatment. - The most immediate and surest remedy is the prohibition of smoking; but often the patient either openly rebels or deceives the doctor; in such cases, only symptomatic treatment can be administered.

Workers in tobacco manufacturing are subject, especially in the beginning, to headaches, nausea, loss of appetite, insomnia, and often diarrhea; *Hurteaux* noted that these symptoms are more pronounced and more frequent in women than in men. In addition, other more or less serious nervous disorders, chronic bronchitis, and chronic skin diseases often occur, which, after a certain time, are associated with a particular cachectic state. In some cases, the skin takes on a dirty gray color, so that an experienced eye could, to a certain extent, recognize those who work with tobacco; but, according to *Hurteaux,* it takes at least two years for this characteristic tint to manifest.

The most obvious indication would be to abandon the

manufacturing process. For tremors and dizziness, strong vinegar inhalations and ammonia liquor (10-15 drops per day) are recommended, purely palliative remedies.

Alcoholic Beverages

Acute Alcoholism. - Acute alcoholism is determined by the introduction into the body of a more or less considerable quantity of alcoholic beverages (wine, beer, absinthe, spirits). While small doses of alcohol have a tonic and healthy action and represent a true food that with its combustion saves that of the tissues, large doses on the contrary produce pathological phenomena, a true intoxication, commonly known by the name of drunkenness.

Noteworthy and curious is the case observed by *Coulon*, of a man who was suddenly seized by attacks of acute alcoholism that recurred several times, and which were not at all due to the ingestion of alcohol, but rather to the inhalation of its vapors. This man was assigned to dye fabrics for the manufacture of flowers and subsequently to progressively decolorize them to obtain the different tones necessary, and for this he had to immerse the leaves, dyed with aniline, in an alcohol bath at 40°-50°.

Alcoholics act on the body by progressively paralyzing the brain, the spinal cord, and the medulla oblongata..

Symptoms and Progression. - The first symptom with which intoxication ordinarily manifests is a general sense of well-being. The intellectual faculties are excited, ideas arise more readily, and it becomes easier to express them with words. The drinker forgets his worries, his sorrows, his pains to abandon himself to noisy, talkative, thoughtless, petulant cheerfulness, and sometimes even tender, sentimental, affectionate. He feels a compelling need to move; he fidgets, leaps up, gesticulates animatedly, jokes, bellows, laughs immoderately, has a special predilection for obscene songs; at the same time, he is still fully aware of his actions and makes every effort to control himself. On the contrary, the individual who "has the bad wine" becomes taciturn, gloomy, the most innocent joke offends him, he is quarrelsome, vindictive, ready to pass from insults to physical altercations.

In the second stage of intoxication, especially when the drinking continues, or when the dose of alcohol ingested at the beginning was strong enough, intelligence soon becomes clouded, ideas become confused and incoherent, intellectual faculties weaken, reason is lost, passions are unleashed with all their vehemence and sometimes drive the drunk to manic acts, to crime, or to suicide. Sensory disturbances arise (amblyopia, diplopia, ringing in the ears, sometimes complete anesthesia); speech becomes difficult and slurred, the gait is staggering, maintaining balance requires immense effort, falls are frequent. The face is red, the eyes appear injected and shiny, the neck veins turgid; sometimes delirium and convulsions appear, but more often a state of invincible drowsiness follows, leading to a deep sleep that lasts several hours and leaves behind a headache, heaviness of head, anorexia, nausea and vomiting, intense thirst, prostration. In severe cases, drowsiness is soon followed by coma, with complete loss of consciousness, anesthesia, weak and slow pulse, vomiting, stertorous breathing, skin cold, pale or cyanotic, covered in a sticky sweat. This state (apoplexy of drinkers) ordinarily lasts two or three days and can end in death due to cerebral hemorrhage or cardiac paralysis; in other cases, the individual is struck by hemiplegia.

Through the ingestion of an exaggerated quantity of alcohol (it is almost always about spirits and non-alcoholic individuals) a severe intoxication can occur, with an extremely acute progression; the drunk collapses as if struck by lightning into a profound coma and death occurs in half an hour or an hour, sometimes after twelve or fifteen hours.

Children are very intolerant of alcohol and often succumb to even small doses administered by imprudent people.

In adolescents, the first period of excitement is usually very short; often convulsions ensue, usually followed by death.

Drunkenness from Beer. - Since beers generally contain little alcohol (2-5%), rather significant quantities are required to produce intoxication; but this is heavier, more serious, more dangerous than that caused by wine.

In the stage of excitement, cheerfulness is very spontaneous and communicative; rather, a state of stupidity, of intellectual stupor is observed, rapidly followed by drowsiness and then by a heavy sleep, which leaves behind an intense headache and a rather persistent general malaise. Moreover, beer often contains toxic substances that can singularly modify the effects produced by alcohol; thus, glycerin, as results from the research of *Dujardin-*

Beaumetz, can provoke convulsions and paralysis; picrotoxin, the alkaloid of the Levant's nut, paralysis and, in habitual abuse, paraplegia.

Harmful effects can also be produced by nux vomica and the lactic acid contained in considerable proportion in some types of beer.

Intoxication from spirits and liqueurs. - Characterized by the rapidity with which symptoms appear and their peculiar severity. Due to the enormous amount of alcohol they contain (rum can contain up to 70 percent), they exert a very powerful and detrimental effect on the brain.

Intoxication from absinthe (*Acute absinthism*). - Here, the harmful effects of alcohol are compounded by those of absinthin. The main symptoms of this intoxication include: muscle tremors and spasms, dizziness, melancholic or frightening hallucinations, a sense of severe malaise, precordial anxiety, and insomnia.

In severe cases, true epileptiform seizures may be observed.

Anatomical lesions of acute alcoholism. - Congestion of the cerebral meninges and brain substance, more pronounced on the upper surface of the brain; the subarachnoid spaces and cerebral ventricles are the site of serous, sometimes bloody, effusions. The lungs are usually congested, edematous, and may also present hemorrhages. Sometimes signs of acute gastroenteritis can also be found. The blood is dark; all organs exude the characteristic odor of alcohol.

Treatment of acute alcoholism. - Emetics should be administered first to promptly evacuate the poison, and stimulants (black coffee, camphor, ammonia - 5-10 drops in half a glass of water or in a cup of coffee) and in more severe cases, hypodermic injections of strychnine (1 centigram at a time; maximum daily dose: 6-7 centigrams).

Against cerebral congestion, cold compresses on the head, mustard plasters on the legs, purgative enemas are to be prescribed; moreover, the patient should lie with their head rather elevated. In the threat of asphyxiation, recourse should be had to cold showers on the head, faradization, inhalations of oxygen, artificial respiration and, if necessary, tracheotomy.

Chronic alcoholism. - The habitual abuse of alcoholics (especially liqueurs) gradually produces a particular pathological state called chronic alcoholism. It is known that ethyl alcohol is much less harmful to the organism than that extracted from beetroots, grain, etc.; this explains why alcoholism is much more frequent and takes a more serious form in the less affluent social classes, especially among the working class, which tend to consume a great deal of wine and other alcohols of lower quality.

It was estimated that the number of people who die each year as victims of alcohol reaches 50,000 in England and exceeds 100,000 in Russia.

Symptoms and course. - After the abuse of alcohol for a more or less extended time, and after repeated bouts of acute alcoholism, disorders of motility begin to appear, consisting mostly of muscular tremors more pronounced in the hands and arms, in the morning when getting up, following new and copious drinking, and in a fasting state. In the case observed by *Hammond,* the individual could hold nothing in their hands unless they fixed them with their gaze; as soon as they stopped looking, the object would fall to the ground. The muscles of the legs, tongue, and speech are in turn affected; the gait becomes uncertain, staggering, and in some cases impossible; speech is difficult and slurred.

In some cases, contractures, muscle spasms, and convulsive seizures are also observed.

Disturbances of sensitivity mainly consist of tingling sensations or piercing pains in the extremities, hyperesthesia and cutaneous anesthesia, which progresses from the extremities towards the central parts and may also be limited to one lateral half of the body (hemianesthesia). The sensory organs generally do not remain unscathed; disturbances of vision (sparkling scotomas, amblyopia) are common, less frequent are those of hearing, taste, and smell. Digestion is deeply disturbed, symptoms of chronic gastroenteric catarrh are noted, with loss of appetite, nausea, vomiting usually in the morning (vomitus matutinus potatorum) watery, generally alkaline, made up largely of swallowed saliva. A consequence of dyspepsia is progressive weight loss (cachexia potatorum) that can reach severe marasmus; with an earthy yellow tint of the skin. The intelligence of the drinker also soon suffers from the pernicious influence of alcohol; apathy, inertia, and intellectual stupor are mostly noted, along with insomnia, nightmares, mostly frightening hallucinations. Rarely the hallucination is of a pleasant nature, although cases have been observed. *Huss* reports that one of his patients saw every day, at noon, a table covered with the most appetizing dishes and the finest wines; happily, he would prepare to sit at the table, but the vision disappeared. Some patients do not remember their hallucinations, others recall them and laugh about it, while others are fully convinced of their reality.

As the disease progresses, strength diminishes increasingly, and physical and moral wasting sometimes reaches the highest degree. When the alcoholic does not die marasmic, they die demented and from general paralysis.

Among the numerous and varied organic alterations that can occur in the course of chronic alcoholism, chronic endocarditis, the callous degeneration of the heart (sclerosis of the coronary arteries), hypertrophy, idiopathic dilatation and fatty degeneration of the heart, tachycardia, arteriosclerosis (atheromatous arteries), chronic pharyngitis, gastrectasis, hemorrhoids; active hyperemia, hypertrophy and fatty infiltration of the liver, liver cirrhosis, chronic indurative pancreatitis, chronic bronchial catarrh, cystitis, and chronic nephritis deserve special mention.

Absinthism constitutes a special variety of chronic alcoholism. This dire habit, fortunately rare in our country, is very widespread in France and especially in America. The symptoms consist essentially of disorders of sensitivity, insomnia, cramps, muscular tremors, nightmares, diminished intellectual and moral faculties, and brutishness associated with severe physical wasting. Hallucinations and convulsive attacks akin to epileptic (absinthic epilepsy) or hysterical fits are common, presenting in two stages:

in the first, generally short, tetanic rigidity of the trunk and neck muscles occurs, causing true opisthotonos (*Lancereaux*); in the second stage, there are disordered convulsions of the limbs with a tendency to bite and tear at the chest. Afterwards, a relative calm is noted, after which the contractions and convulsions reappear; the attack usually lasts about an hour.

While alcoholism causes anesthesia, especially at the extremities of the limbs, absinthism causes hyperesthesia that extends to the trunk, so that compressing the lower anterior region of the abdomen produces phenomena similar to those observed by pressing the ovary in hysterical women.

Anatomical lesions of chronic alcoholism include congestion of the cerebral meninges and brain; pachymeningitis sometimes hemorrhagic. The stomach, in addition to the symptoms of chronic catarrh, may show significant thickening of its walls and sometimes perforating ulcers. In the parenchymatous organs (liver, kidneys, lungs, etc.), there is usually chronic interstitial inflammation or fatty degeneration.

The vessels may be the site of various alterations (endarteritis, atheromatosis, thrombosis, aneurysms, etc.).

Treatment of chronic alcoholism involves the suppression of alcoholic beverages, prescription of hydrotherapy, the use of strychnine in progressively increasing doses until maximum tolerance, abstinence from smoking and sexual intercourse. Against tremors, Paul recommends electric baths. Observations by a Russian physician, *Skvorizow*, seem to indicate that tincture of strophanthus can rapidly alleviate attacks of dipsomania.

It was by chance that he noticed this curious property of

the medicine in question: he was treating an obese 63-year-old man who, being in full dipsomaniac crisis, drank incessantly large amounts of spirits. Since the patient presented weakness and intermittency of the pulse, he deemed it necessary to raise cardiac action with tincture of strophanthus, at a dose of 7 drops 3 times a day. From the first dose, the patient was seized by nausea and developed such a disgust for alcohol that he abruptly and permanently stopped its use.

Prophylaxis is of great importance. The law must impose and ensure the absolute rectification of all alcohol so that no impure alcohol or alcoholic beverage can be placed on the market. Elementary courses in hygiene must be held in schools, highlighting the terrible consequences of the abuse of alcoholic beverages. The authority must prevent the preparation and sale of products harmful to health; it is up to private initiative to open premises where only hygienic beverages are sold. Frequent sanitary inspections must also be ordered to examine the nature of the alcohol that is put on the market.

Delirium tremens. - Among the mental afflictions due to chronic alcoholism, "delirium tremens" (alcoholic delirium, alcoholic madness), as *Lancereaux* says, is nothing but an acute and accidental episode of chronic alcoholism. The causes that can determine the development of an attack of trembling delirium are alcoholic excesses or the abrupt suppression of the habitual intoxicant, certain febrile diseases (typhus, pneumonia, erysipelas, scarlet fever, acute articular rheumatism, etc.), traumatic injuries, emotional upheavals. Sometimes it is also observed after a long time of abstaining from drinking, as in prisoners confined for several years.

Symptoms of the attack. - Rarely does this delirium burst forth suddenly; in the majority of cases, it follows various psychic disturbances (nightmares, visual hallucinations, insomnia, etc.). The onset of the attack is characterized by the patient's incessant loquacity, by a great restlessness, a need to move, to walk, by a tremor of the limbs that is more or less considerable but neither general nor persistent, insomnia, stubborn constipation, oliguria, and an absence of fever. Hallucinations are at the core of delirium tremens. Initially, the patient sees objects as if through a fog; then gradually, they begin to see trembling objects, fluttering red cloths, sparks, flames moving in all directions continuously; at other times, they see threatening specters, monsters with gaping mouths ready to devour them, animals with fiery eyes, rats, snakes, cats appearing and scurrying everywhere, armed men, battles, massacres, fires that throw them into the most cruel fright.

Auditory hallucinations at first consist of buzzes, whispers, hisses, soon followed by more distinct noises: bells, sobs, cries, screams, moans, curses, threats; often, the hallucinated individual believes they can distinguish among these various noises the voices of known people.

Hallucinations of taste, smell, and touch can also be observed: foods and drinks have horrible flavors; the room smells of corpses; the skin is pricked by myriads of insects, worms crawl under the skin, threads constricting from all sides. The patient's face, so to speak, reflects the nature of these hallucinations; now contorted with terror, anger, fury, now with melancholy, despair; sometimes the hallucinated person is driven to manic acts, lunging at those nearby, or attempting suicide.

These episodes of delirium typically last only a few days, then gradually disappear, and recovery can be complete; in other cases, there are more or less numerous relapses, the patient becomes hypochondriacal or tormented by vague ideas of persecution.

Febrile delirium tremens. - In this form, the tremor extends to all the muscles of the body and does not disappear during sleep. A careful examination reveals small undulations produced by the alternate lifting of superficial muscle bundles; by applying the hand, one can also feel the small shocks that agitate the deep muscles.

When this state persists, the patient rapidly progresses to nervous exhaustion and muscular weakness, and in this state of incomplete paralysis, which mainly affects the lower limbs, death usually ensues (*Vétault*).

Treatment. - The patient must be isolated in a quiet and dark room, and sleep must be induced with opium (0.10 every 3 hours), with morphine, with pure chloral hydrate or combined with morphine. To avoid collapse, alcoholic beverages must be permitted, and cold affusion baths, hypodermic injections of strychnine may also be useful. According to *Russell,* the best means to combat delirium effectively and safely and swiftly is trional, which should be preferred over all other hypnotics in these cases; its use does not cause any sort of accident.

Krafft-Ebing strongly recommends the use of methylal (1-4

grams in a 150-gram potion). Paraldehyde also proves effective (3 grams in orange flower water).

Ether.

Ethyl ether (sulfuric ether [C²H³] ²O) is obtained by reacting sulfuric acid with alcohol at high temperature. It is a colorless liquid, highly volatile, extremely flammable, with a characteristic odor and a burning taste.

When inhaled, it produces anesthesia; when ingested, it is absorbed and eliminated by the body much more quickly than alcohol, promptly causing transient intoxication, usually followed by deep sleep with anesthesia.

"Ether drinkers" are numerous in the northern regions of America and Europe (Ireland); the ether consumed is the commercial kind, which pharmacists and liquor dealers sell at the price of ten cents for a dose of 10-15 grams. Since this liquid is very light, it is possible there to poison oneself quite cheaply.

According to *Huart*, in those regions everyone drinks ether, men and women, adults and children. The average dose is 10 grams at a time, and this is repeated two, three, or even six times during the day. Some swallow it neat, those who are less accustomed drink water first, and then the ether. The effects that follow almost immediately upon its absorption are much like those produced by alcohol, yet they are distinguished by a much greater rapidity. Over time, when poisoning has become habitual, other symptoms arise: epileptiform convulsions and mania.

Ether does not produce serious organic lesions like alcohol; it passes almost without leaving a trace, and moderate drinkers enjoy good health, at most complaining of dyspepsia. Heavy drinkers, on the other hand, suffer from weakness, neurasthenia, muscular tremors. Some concede that habitual abuse of ether can lead to mental alienation, others deny it; however, it has long been universally recognized that the use of this intoxicant shortens life.

Chloroform (Trichloromethane, CHCl³).

Chloroform is a colorless, very clear liquid with an initially pungent taste, then fresh and sweet. It has a very pleasant ethereal odor, is slightly soluble in water, which it endows with a pleasant and sweet taste.

Here we do not intend to discuss the accidents that sometimes occur in chloroform anesthesia performed in serious surgical operations, but rather the phenomena that occur following the ingestion of this substance. The toxic dose is highly variable; 4 grams can cause poisoning, in other cases recovery occurred even after ingesting more than 60 grams. In a case observed by *Jackson* and reported by *Taylor*, a man who had swallowed 150 grams of chloroform recovered after five days, although the symptoms that appeared were very severe.

Symptoms and course of poisoning. - A few minutes after ingestion, a sort of drunkenness occurs, associated with dizziness and confusion of ideas, promptly followed by coma and complete loss of consciousness. The pupils are dilated, the pulse is weak and slow, the breathing is stertorous, the temperature is lowered, the body is shaken by convulsions; death can occur within a few hours due to cardiac paralysis. More often, however, after some time the poisoned person wakes up from their stupor, vomiting appears, and a slow and gradual improvement is observed; however, throat and abdominal pains, cough, and sometimes jaundice remain for a few days.

Anatomical lesions. - The mucous membrane of the stomach and the first part of the intestine is sometimes hyperemic and inflamed. The lungs, and rarely also the brain, are heavily congested. The heart is flabby and contains dark and fluid blood. The corpse exhales the characteristic odor of chloroform.

Treatment. - Stimulants (coffee, camphor, strychnine; *Kœppen* recommends picrotoxin); skin revulsants. Artificial respiration.

Chloral (C^2Cl^3OH).

Chloral, discovered in 1832 by *Liebig*, is obtained by acting chlorine on alcohol. It is a colorless liquid, oily in appearance and to the touch, with a sharp and irritating odor, similar to that of chloroform, and an acrid, caustic, bitter, and aromatic taste. It is extremely soluble in water, alcohol, and ether. With the addition of a small amount of water, it heats up and gives rise to a solid, crystalline mass: chloral hydrate (C^2HCl^3O, H^2O), a substance highly soluble in water.

A few grams of chloral can already produce symptoms of intoxication; a dose of 2 and a half grams was sometimes fatal for children.

Symptoms. - They are generally observed following ingestion of rather high doses of this substance, 15-20 grams or more (it is almost always suicides or attempted suicides), and have much in common with the symptoms of opium and morphine poisoning, and consist mainly in deep sopor with very obvious constriction of the pupils, loss of consciousness, complete anesthesia, cooling of the extremities, abolition of reflex activity, complete relaxation of muscles and sphincters, very weak, laborious, stertorous breathing, deep collapse in which death often supervenes.

Sometimes, instead of these depressive phenomena, a violent, furious delirium sets in, with more or less generalized tetanic shocks. Death occurs due to progressive respiratory embarrassment, or cardiac paralysis.

Treatment. - Emetics, gastric lavage. Stimulants strychnine, caffeine, etc. Atropine is administered as an antagonist to chloral; *Falck* reports that a woman attempted poisoning with 20-24 grams of chloral hydrate, and the doctors, assuming morphine poisoning, injected 1 and a half milligrams of atropine, following which the pulse rose and the other phenomena gradually dissipated only the following morning. According to *Kæppen's* experimental research, picrotoxin raises the activity of the respiratory and circulatory centers in chloral-induced narcosis.

It is necessary to prevent the patient from cooling by

wrapping them in warm woolen blankets, placing hot water bottles, heated bricks at their feet, and also heating the room.

Benzene (C^6H^6)

It is a clear, colorless liquid, with a universally known ethereal odor, commonly and very frequently used; it affects the organism like alcohols, mainly causing paralysis of the brain.

The ingestion of this hydrocarbon, in toxic doses, leads to stupor, dizziness, convulsive attacks, impotence, coma, loss of consciousness, as well as various disturbances of intelligence: hallucinations, delirium, speech confusion which can go as far as aphasia. In some cases, cyanosis of the face and extremities, anemia, and circulatory disorders were also noted.

Factory workers involved with gasoline production and those frequently using this substance often present with anemia, paresis, paralysis, anesthesia, hyperesthesia, and sexual weakness (*Quinquaud*).

Treatment includes gastric lavage, emetics, stimulants, and artificial respiration.

Quinine (Cinchona).

The trees providing quinine belong to the "cinchona"

genus and the Rubiaceae family; the main species are Cinchona officinalis and C. calisaya. They are native to South America, especially Peru, Bolivia, and Brazil.

These beautiful and elegant trees can grow over 20 meters tall; their bark, when pulverized, constitutes the commercial quinine. It contains various alkaloids, of which the most important is quinine ($C^{20}H^{24}N^2O^2+nH^2O$), which appears as a crystallized substance in small, silky needles. It is odorless, very bitter, alkaline, almost insoluble in cold water, soluble in alcohol and ether, and forms with acids crystallized salts which, in solution, exhibit characteristic opalescence.

Therapeutic doses of quinine (1-2 grams) produce dizziness, confusion, drowsiness (quinine intoxication), ringing, buzzing in the ears with hypoacusis, and sometimes temporary deafness, visual disturbances: photophobia, and amblyopia. Trousseau observed a case of transient madness in a nun from only 1 gram and 25 centigrams of quinine sulfate taken at once.

Larger doses (3 grams) usually cause headaches, vertigo, facial pallor, dilated pupils with pupil immobility, amblyopia, and sometimes complete blindness and deafness, as in a case observed in an adult by *Trousseau*. The pulse is very weak and slowed; delirium ensues followed by deep coma and loss of consciousness. The sense of color is restored later than vision; the visual field after the disappearance of amaurosis remains concentrically restricted.

If the dose is even higher (4-8 grams), death can occur due to cardiac and respiratory paralysis; in cases of recovery, and also in cases of overly prolonged quinine treatments, deafness often persists for years and perhaps for a lifetime. This deafness is caused by chronic congestion of the tympanic membrane.

Cantani reports the case of a young man deaf for 11 years following a prolonged quinine treatment prescribed at the age of 5 for intermittent fever. *Miling* observed mutism lasting over a year in a twelve-year-old child. Lurini and Bortoluzzi were able to observe fatal cases of tetanus developing after hypodermic injections of quinine.

The treatment is symptomatic.

Antipyrine ($C_{11}H_{12}N_2O$).

Antipyrine is a crystalline powder, white or grayish-red in color, with an initially piquant and bitter taste, though not as strong as that of quinine or as lingering. It is soluble in ether and very soluble in water.

Antipyrine is rapidly absorbed through the digestive tract; in some instances, severe "shock" incidents and even fatal poisonings have occurred from relatively small doses (0.40 to 2 grams).

Its toxic action primarily affects the nervous centers, inducing paralysis without prior excitation (*Arduin* and *Coppola*).

Symptoms. - In mild cases, symptoms consist of nausea, vomiting, epigastric pain, diarrhea, transient skin rashes (erythema, roseola, urticaria with intense skin itching), and profuse sweating, sometimes accompanied by symptoms of psychic excitation.

In severe cases, there is a decrease in temperature, profuse sweating, digestive disturbances, oliguria, distress, dizziness, extreme weakness with a tendency toward syncope, temporary amaurosis, weak cardiac contractions, small, irregular, and intermittent pulse, dyspnea, stupor, coma; death may ensue in this state.

Other times, there may be tremors, contractions of the facial muscles, tetanic or epileptiform convulsions followed by profound coma. Hemorrhages have also been rarely observed (epistaxis, ecchymoses, purpura, metrorrhagia, hemoptysis).

Treatment. - Prevention involves starting with small doses (0.50 grams) of the medication and only increasing this dose when it is well-tolerated.

In cases of poisoning, atropine should be administered; sodium bicarbonate has been useful against gastric pains and vomiting in many cases.

Carbon Dioxide (CO2)
(Carbonic acid, carbonic anhydride, mofette, must air, etc.).

This colorless, odorless gas is produced by combustion, fermentation, and in coal mines. It can be simply mixed with air or result from the consumption of oxygen in enclosed spaces, especially in small or poorly ventilated rooms.

Poisonings by carbon dioxide are not uncommon; it is well-known as a means often used by those committing suicide.

Death is not due to a directly toxic action like that of carbon monoxide, but rather to a lack of oxygen; however, similar anesthesia phenomena produced by chloroform are observed.

Symptoms of poisoning. - When inhaled pure or mixed with a small amount of atmospheric air, this gas can cause sneezing, violent coughing, glottis spasm, and rapid death by suffocation if the individual is not immediately moved to fresh air. When the proportion of carbon dioxide in the air is lower (40-60:100), there is initially a feeling of heaviness in the head and pressure at the temples, ringing in the ears, sometimes vomiting, drowsiness, dizziness, muscular weakness, and then an inability to move, loss of sensation, delirium, and hallucinations, deep coma, death. Breathing, at first difficult and stertorous, ultimately becomes more and more dyspneic; the heartbeats, very violent at first, become progressively weaker and then cease.

Anatomical lesions. - Blood stasis and hyperemia in the brain, heart, lungs, and many other organs; occasionally, ecchymoses are found on the mucosa of the digestive tract. The blood is black, thick, fluid; bright red if death occurred due to carbon dioxide produced by combustion.

Treatment. - The asphyxiated person must be immediately moved to open air; skin revulsives (mustard plasters on the chest, etc.); cold showers on the head and chest; artificial respiration. Stimulants. Inhalation of oxygen. In the most serious cases, blood transfusion.

Illuminating Gas

The gas used for illumination usually consists of dihydrogen carbide, hydrogen, and carbon monoxide.

Many cases of poisoning, especially accidental ones due to illuminating gas, have been diligently observed and reported; however, *Pettenkofer* believes that perhaps an even greater number of these cases remain unknown. A physician in Augsburg was treating a patient for "typhoid fever," and would have continued this treatment if a lady with an extremely delicate sense of smell had not discovered and reported a small gas leak, thus saving the patient's life.

At other times, the gas that poisons the air of a room or an apartment comes from pipes that pass at a certain distance from the house, as in the interesting case observed by *Guillié* and reported by *Brouardel*. The poisoned individuals had no gas lines in their ground-floor accommodations; the line was hidden in the street, in a trench 80 centimeters deep, parallel to the houses and 1.8 meters away from them. After a gas leak, approximately 100 cubic meters of gas filtered through the soil of two small houses, especially into one that was poorly paved. Of the six people who breathed this gas in varying amounts during their sleep due to the different nature of the locations, one died after four days, completely unconscious, and the other five recovered quite quickly, although two were seriously poisoned. *Brouardel* notes that in cases of poisoning by illuminating gas from a distance, explosions never occur, and that in the case in question there were none, although a lamp had been kept lit in the victims' houses, and that moreover, the characteristic smell of illuminating gas is never perceived in these conditions. This lack of detonation and smell is due to the fact that among the various gases that make up the illuminating gas, carbon monoxide, an odorless gas contained in the proportion of 8-9:100, filters through the soil more easily than the others.

The penetration of gas from the soil into houses was also noted at a distance of 54 meters from where the pipe break occurred. According to *Eulenberg* and *Pokrowscky*, 5:100 of illuminating gas mixed with the air we breathe is sufficient to produce fatal effects in humans.

Symptoms of poisoning. - They are very similar to those produced by carbon monoxide. Initially headache, dizziness, nausea with vomiting, pressure at the temples, ringing in the ears, and flashes before the eyes; subsequently, loss of consciousness, cyanosis of the skin, general depression, convulsions, paralysis, death with symptoms of asphyxia.

As after-effects, in cases where the poisoned individual was timely rescued, paralysis is most often observed; disturbances of sensitivity and speech, etc.

The treatment is the same as for carbon monoxide poisoning or other asphyxiations.

V - Paralyzing Poisons
of the peripheral nerves and muscles.

Curare.

Curare (also known as curari, urari, woorara) comes to us from the Amazon River, the banks of the Orinoco, the Guianas, and Peru in small clay pots with a parchment-covered opening at the top. It is a poison used by the natives of South America to poison their arrows and appears as a syrupy or solid extract, black, with a glass-like fracture, an empyreumatic odor, and a very bitter taste. It is insoluble in ether, partially soluble in alcohol, chloroform, and water. This very potent poison is a mixture of various other plant and animal toxins.

The active principle of curare is an alkaloid isolated in 1865 by *Preyer.*

According to *Claude Bernard,* curarine ($C^{10}H^{15}N$) would have an action quite similar to that of curare, but would be about twenty times more active than the curare from which it was extracted. This alkaloid is crystallizable, deliquescent; with mineral acids, it can form crystallizable salts. 1 milligram of this substance, administered by subcutaneous injection, kills a rabbit.

Curare can be ingested with impunity at a dose eighty times higher than what would be lethal by subcutaneous injection or direct inoculation into the bloodstream because it is eliminated by the kidneys as it enters the blood from the digestive tract, and consequently cannot accumulate in sufficient quantity to cause poisoning.

As extensively demonstrated by the experiments of *Claude Bernard*, curare acts by paralyzing the terminal plates of the motor nerves, reducing the conductivity of sensory nerves and the reflex power of the spinal cord, paralyzing the vagus nerve, and causing a decrease in temperature.

Symptoms of poisoning. - These are those of a progressive weakening until complete paralysis of both voluntary and reflex movements, with a decrease in temperature and death due to respiratory paralysis.

Treatment. - If the poison has been absorbed through a wound or sore, a local application of phenic acid, sodium chloride, or potassium iodide will be made; sucking the wound or applying cups, and performing stimulating and warm rubs will also be useful; diuretics will be administered at the same time to eliminate the poison more promptly. If the toxin has been ingested, a good emetic will be given; artificial respiration may prevent the danger of asphyxia.

Aconitum napellus (*Aconitum napellus*, L.)

This plant, belonging to the Ranunculaceae family, thrives in the shady places of mountains and hills and is also cultivated for ornamentation in our gardens; it blooms in May and June. It has smooth, alternate leaves divided into 5 or 7 elongated, deeply jagged lobes. The flowers are large, blue, hermaphroditic,

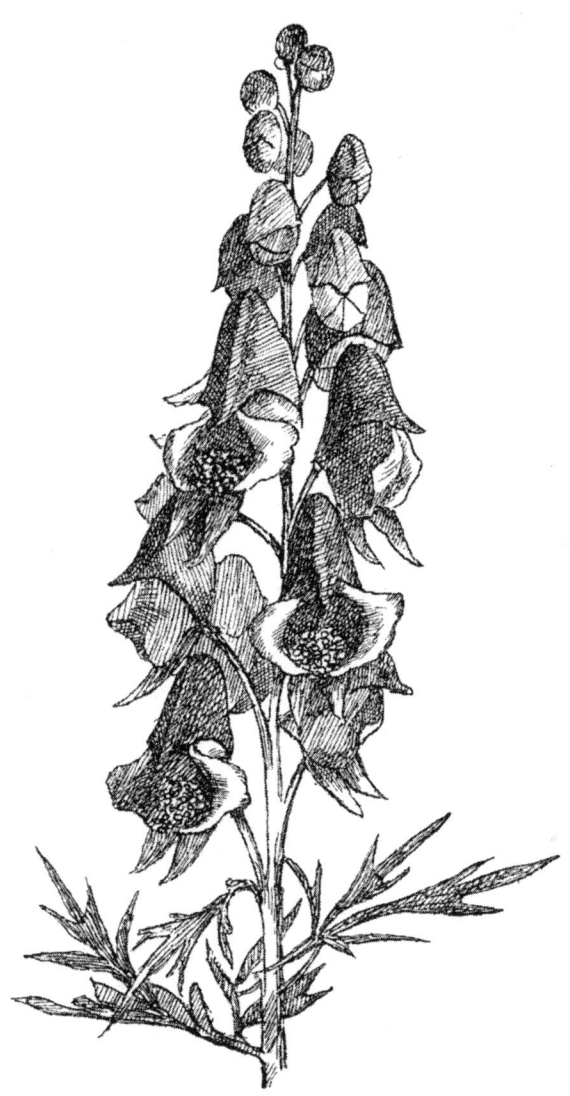

somewhat pedunculated; they form a cluster about 30 centimeters long; they have a calyx made up of 5 unequal petaloid sepals: one upper, more developed, in the shape of a concave hood on the bottom; two lateral ones flat, rounded, hairy on their inner face; two lower, somewhat smaller, oval, also hairy on their inner face. The corolla consists of 2 clawed petals, straight, ending at the top with a sort of small hood and hidden under the upper sepal. All parts of the plant, especially the leaves and the root, are poisonous.

The plant's active principle, discovered by *Brandes,* is aconitine ($C_{30}H_{47}NO_7$), a brownish, brittle alkaloid that easily reduces to a yellowish-white powder, very soluble in ether and alcohol, slightly soluble in water, with a very acrid taste. It is one of the most potent toxins known; a dose of 4-5 milligrams can be lethal for an adult.

Other species of aconite used for preparing various medicines or for extracting alkaloids are: "aconitum heterophyllum" (atis, atus of the Indians), "aconitum ferox" (bish or bikh of the Indians), more active than napellus, "aconitum anthora", "aconitum lycoctonum", indigenous, highly poisonous, rich in picrotoxin..

Aconite poisonings are usually accidental; sometimes the root of this plant was mistakenly exchanged for that of horseradish; in other cases, the tincture of aconite intended for external use was ingested. *Bouchardat* relates the case of twelve individuals who, suffering from pellagra and scurvy, mistakenly took 90 grams each of aconite juice instead of cochlearia juice. A 60-year-old man first showed symptoms of severe poisoning and died within minutes; two elderly women died in two hours, the other nine suffered serious accidents, and were with great difficulty saved from death. *Willis* observed the case of a man who died manically in a very short time for having eaten a salad in which fresh aconite leaves were found. There are also cases of criminal poisonings carried out with powdered aconite root, or with the tincture.

Aconite paralyzes the peripheral terminals of the motor nerves like curare, produces a special modification of the sensitive innervation, whose effects are especially felt in the trigeminal area; it also paralyzes the respiratory muscles and causes the heart to stop.

Symptoms of poisoning. - Shortly after ingesting the poison, a burning sensation in the mouth is felt, and symptoms of toxic gastroenteritis appear, with severe nervous symptoms: tingling, anesthesia of the tongue and fingers of the hands and feet, headache, dizziness, amaurosis, deafness, aphasia, facial neuralgia, drowsiness. The pulse is slow, the breathing dyspnoeic, the skin livid, covered with cold sweats; violent cramps usually occur with anesthesia and complete loss of consciousness; death can occur within a few hours.

Vibert and *Lhotte* had occasion to observe multiple poisonings caused by the unintentional substitution of aconitine tincture for quinine tincture in the preparation of a quinine wine. Six people drank, at different times, a liqueur glass of this wine, and three of them took it twice, morning and evening; three died after a few hours, and the others were more or less seriously poisoned. In all these cases, the same symptoms were noted: after a quarter of an hour or half an hour from ingestion, general malaise, tingling and prickling in the mouth, numbness of the tongue and lips, vomiting, and finally a sense of general cooling with a tendency to syncope; they had neither convulsions, visual disturbances, nor complete loss of consciousness.

In fatal cases, the autopsy found the heart stopped in diastole, the blood dark, asphyctic, and strong congestion of the brain and digestive tract.

Treatment. - No antidotes are known; stomach emptying and the administration of tannin or tannic preparations, and atropine are recommended. Symptomatic treatment.

Hemlock (*Cicuta major, Conium maculatum*, L.)

This plant, belonging to the Umbelliferae family, has a biennial, fusiform, taproot, with an herbaceous, straight, branched, 1-2 meters tall, glabrous, cylindrical, glaucous, somewhat striated stem marked with dark purple spots. The leaves are alternate, very large, tripinnate, with long, deeply serrated leaflets. The flowers are small, white, arranged in terminal umbels. The greater hemlock grows in waste and stony places, along the less-traveled paths of villages; it blooms in June and July.

The *lesser hemlock* (*Aethusa cynapium*, L.) is very similar to the greater hemlock, but its herbaceous stem is less tall; it grows in cultivated places, gardens, near old walls; it blooms in July..

The *water hemlock* (Cicuta virosa) has a large and fleshy root, a straight, branched, hollow stem, 60 centimeters to 1 meter tall. Its leaves, especially the lower ones, are very large, tripinnate; its flowers closely resemble those of the greater hemlock. It grows on the banks of streams and ponds and is more poisonous than the former; the effects it causes are more severe and intense..

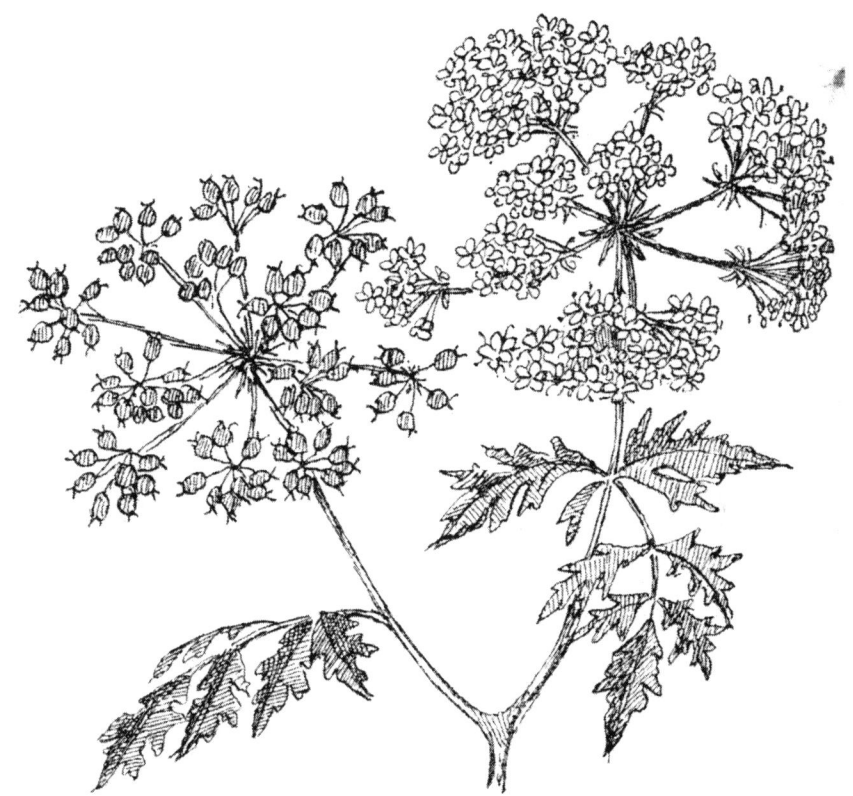

The toxic principle of these plants is coniine or cicutoxin ($C^8H^{17}N$), an oily, yellowish liquid, slightly soluble in water, very soluble in alcohol and ether, with a sharp and unpleasant smell, and a pungent and caustic taste. With sulfuric, phosphoric, nitric, and oxalic acids, it forms compounds that crystallize in large prisms. A dose of 2 decigrams can cause death in humans in a few moments; a single drop can cause severe symptoms of poisoning.

Poisoning by hemlock can be accidental or criminal; it usually involves an overdose of medicinal doses, especially of hemlock extract, the application of hemlock plasters on sores and wounds, or the ingestion of leaves or roots, mistaken for parsley leaves or parsnip roots.

It is believed that some birds, such as larks and quails, are resistant to the toxic properties of hemlock, so much so that they could feed on this plant without any inconvenience; however, their flesh in these cases becomes impregnated with such an amount of toxin that it would suffice to poison anyone who ate it.

Criminal poisonings have been noted following the administration of hemlock infusions or soups containing leaves or roots of this plant.

Hemlock is a paralyzing poison; its action on the motor nerves is similar to that of curare, with the difference, however, that coniine paralyzes the nerve endings of the vagus, which curare leaves intact (*Vulpian*); sensitivity is less affected than motility, it undergoes only a mild and progressive weakening. The brain is usually immune, and intelligence remains intact.

Symptoms of poisoning. - They arise quickly, within an hour, and sometimes even earlier. There is intense headache, dizziness, staggering and uncertain gait, and shortly after a sense of dryness in the mouth with intense thirst, sometimes impossible swallowing, nausea, vomiting, and diarrhea. Visual disturbances occur: flashing scotomas, mydriasis, amblyopia or amaurosis, and serious nervous symptoms: convulsions, fainting, sometimes furious delirium, followed by coma (lowering of temperature, small and slow pulse, difficult and stertorous breathing), and usually death by asphyxia within 3-6 hours.

Anatomical lesions. - Livid spots, skin hemorrhages; passive congestion of internal organs and meninges. Disseminated ecchymoses may be found on the gastroenteric mucosa. The blood is black and fluid.

Treatment. - Emetics and purgatives to expel the poison, tannic acid to neutralize it. Stimulants (concentrated coffee, wine, ether, etc.) will be valuable against collapse; in the event of threatening asphyxia, cold effusions and artificial respiration will be used.

Calabar Bean

The Calabar bean is the seed of Physostigma venenosum, a large leguminous plant often reaching twenty meters in height, native to Calabar in the Gulf of Guinea. The seeds are elongated, slightly curved, glabrous, with a leathery coat marked along its entire length by a linear hilum. From these pulverized seeds, physostigmine or eserine ($C^{30}H^{21}N^3O^4$) is extracted, which appears as colorless, bitter, tabular, and rhomboidal crystals, soluble in alcohol, ether, chloroform, and sparingly soluble in water. Physostigmine is essentially impure eserine.

Poisonings from the Calabar bean are usually accidental; two Glasgow girls were slightly poisoned after imprudently eating fragments of these seeds. In 1864, sixty children in Liverpool were poisoned following ingestion of these beans, which they found in the discharge from a ship, the "Commodore," coming from the shores of Calabar; all but one were saved by vomiting.

Symptoms of poisoning. - Following ingestion of the Calabar bean, violent vomiting with intense colic pains, diarrhea, severe general weakness, tremors, and sometimes tetanic convulsions, pupil miosis, and amblyopia quickly ensue; the pulse is small, irregular, very weak, and frequent, dyspnea, increased secretions: profuse sweating, salivation, tearing, polyuria; then motor paralysis progresses from the lower limbs upwards. Consciousness usually remains unchanged; death occurs due to respiratory and cardiac paralysis.

Treatment. - Emetics, gastric lavage. Stimulants (coffee, camphor, ether, etc.), cutaneous revulsives. Artificial respiration.

Ergot (*Secale cornutum*).

Ergot, also known as *sphacelia segetum* or *sclerotium clavus*, is a grain measuring 1-3 centimeters in length, cylindrical, blunt, more or less curved, with a brownish-purple color, an extremely unpleasant smell, and a compact texture. It develops not only on rye but also on corn and other grasses, containing two active substances: ergotamine or ergotoxine and sclerotic acid.

The powder of ergot is grayish, with an acrid and nauseating taste, a particular unpleasant odor; it greases paper and deteriorates very easily.

Ergot resembles veratrum, curare, and the Calabar bean in one aspect of poisoning, for its paralytic form; they are all paralyzing poisons, but some of them affect the muscular tissue like veratrum, the Calabar bean, and ergot, while curare affects the nervous tissue (*Semmola*).

Acute poisoning (acute ergotism) - Generally occurs after the administration of exaggerated doses (over 4 grams) of ergot to provoke abortion, but it can also be observed after the ingestion of bread containing a considerable quantity, as in six cases observed by *Riker*.

The *symptoms* are initially those of a more or less intense gastroenteric inflammation: nausea, vomiting, colic pains, and diarrhea. Later, nervous phenomena also occur: headache, dizziness, pupil dilation, and amblyopia, severe prostration; in rare cases, also neuralgia and disturbances of intelligence. The pulse is very slow.

In the most severe cases, stupor is noted; death occurs in deep coma.

Treatment. - Emetics, purgatives. Tannic acid, iodinated water to neutralize the poison. Stimulants, black coffee, ether, camphor, ammonia. Vegetable lemonades and mucilaginous potions are also useful.

Chronic poisoning (chronic ergotism). - The prolonged use of bread or flours containing ergot can lead to intoxication that can manifest in two forms: the convulsive and the gangrenous. Ergotoxine would be the cause of the convulsions, while the action of sclerotic acid would be responsible for the gangrenous form.

According to *Poehl*, the toxicity of spoiled flours should be attributed to ptomaines that form from the decomposition of peptones coming from the albuminoid substances of the flour. Ergot has the property of transforming albuminoid substances and would thus indirectly contribute to the formation of ptomaines in the flour.

A) **Convulsive form.** - It starts with a tingling sensation in the limbs, accompanied by paresthesia (itching) or even complete cutaneous anesthesia, headache, dizziness, precordial anxiety, fatigue, and severe general malaise.

Very painful muscular cramps then occur, and in severe cases epileptiform convulsions, cataplexy, and even tetanus (opisthotonos); death may occur due to syncope, asphyxia, or collapse.

Treatment. - Antispasmodics, opium, hydrotherapy.

B) **Gangrenous form** - This form also initially presents with headache, dizziness, and a tingling sensation in the limbs, but after some time, the appearance of dry gangrene in the hands and feet is observed. This gangrene is produced by the anemia resulting from thrombotic occlusion of arteries or from the spastic contraction of the arteries and capillaries. The necrotic parts usually end up detaching.

Treatment. - Opium, stimulants, and local antiseptics. Little can be expected from the amputation of gangrenous parts, as it is not a purely local lesion.

VI - Heart Paralytics

Digitalis (*Digitalis purpurea*, L.)

This beautiful scrophulariaceae has a perennial root, a simple, straight stem ranging from 60 centimeters to 1 meter in height, cylindrical and velvety; leaves are petiolate, oval, acuminate, whitish, velvety. The flowers are purple, pedunculated, hanging, and form a long cluster at the upper part of the stem. The calyx is deeply divided into 5 parts, the corolla is irregularly bell-shaped with 5 unequal, short, and blunt lobes, speckled on the inside with small black dots provided with long, soft hairs. It blooms around June, grows naturally in mountain woods, and is also widely cultivated in gardens for the beauty of its flowers. All parts of the plant, but especially the leaves, are poisonous; the active ingredient is a glucoside, digitalin ($C^5H^8O^2$), a bitter substance, slightly soluble in water, very soluble in alcohol, ether, and chloroform. The toxic but not yet lethal dose of digitalin is 16 milligrams according to *Heer*, 30 according to *Leroux,* and 45 according to *Chereau.*

Poisonings from digitalis or digitalin are usually accidental, through ingestion of parts of the plant or too strong doses of pharmaceutical preparations. However, there are also poisonings from suicide, and criminal acts are not absent.

Symptoms of poisoning. - They generally appear after 1-3 hours from ingestion, and sometimes even earlier; in very rare cases, they did not appear until after 24 hours. The patients

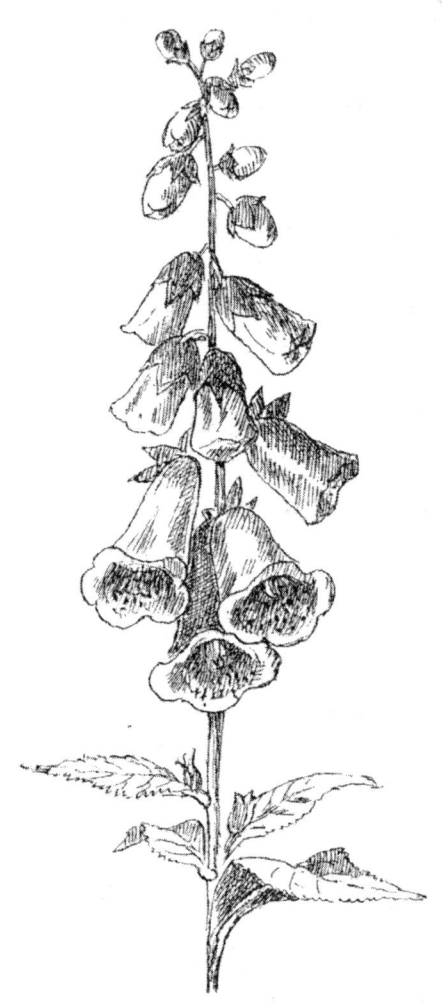

complain of a sense of malaise, dizziness, ringing in the ears, nausea. Shortly thereafter, repeated and violent vomiting, diarrhea, soreness of the gastric region, dyspnea, irregularity and slowing of the pulse, visual disturbances: mydriasis, amblyopia with exophthalmos, then delirium, drowsiness, collapse, and in severe cases death from cardiac paralysis, sometimes within

2-3 days, but usually after 5-10 days. *Barth* reports the case of a woman suffering from anasarca who, following the ingestion of 25 grams of digitalis tincture that had been prescribed for rubbing, died within three-quarters of an hour with no other symptoms than abundant vomiting, general malaise, and very severe pain in the epigastrium.

In non-fatal cases, convalescence is rather slow, and for a while, the patients complain of great weakness, amblyopia, heaviness of the head, and dizziness.

Anatomical lesions. - They are not very characteristic; in addition to the inflammation of the gastro-enteric mucosa, congestion of the liver, and sometimes also of the kidneys and lungs is observed. The heart is flaccid, the right ventricle and the vena cava are engorged with blood.

Treatment. - Emetics, gastric lavage, purgatives. Tannin. Stimulants (camphor, ether, strong coffee, alcohol, ammoniated anise liquor). Cutaneous revulsives (mustard plasters, etc.).

Strophantus (Strophantus hispidus)

This plant is a member of the Apocynaceae family, native to Senegambia and Gabon, where it is used to prepare arrow poison. From its seeds, a glycoside named strophanthin ($C_{31}H_{48}O_{12}$) is extracted, a white substance that is soluble in water and alcohol, insoluble in ether, chloroform, petroleum, and oils.

Strophanthus and strophanthin, as established from

the research by *Polaillon* and *Carville*, act on the organism like digitalis and digitoxin; however, while the latter primarily affects the myocardium and secondarily the heart's nerves, strophanthin (as well as helleborin) is believed to act exclusively on the cardiac muscle, and only transiently on the heart's innervation.

Black Hellebore (*Elleborus niger*, L.)

This plant, belonging to the Ranunculaceae family, grows in most European regions and is low-growing, with long-petioled leaves and pretty pink flowers, solitary or arranged in groups of two or three at the top of a common stem. It is widely cultivated, and due to its blooming period, it is commonly called "Christmas rose".

According to *Wibmer*, the rhizome shows the greatest activity, but the leaves, used in an infusion, are also very toxic: the active principles are two glycosides, helleborin, and helleborein.

Symptoms of poisoning include those of a violent gastroenteritis, with slowed circulation and respiration, a drop in temperature, nephritis (albuminuria, hematuria), mydriasis, headache, delirium, and sometimes death amid convulsions or in stupor due to respiratory arrest and cardiac paralysis.

Treatment involves emetics, gastric lavage. Tannin or tannic preparations. Symptomatic care.

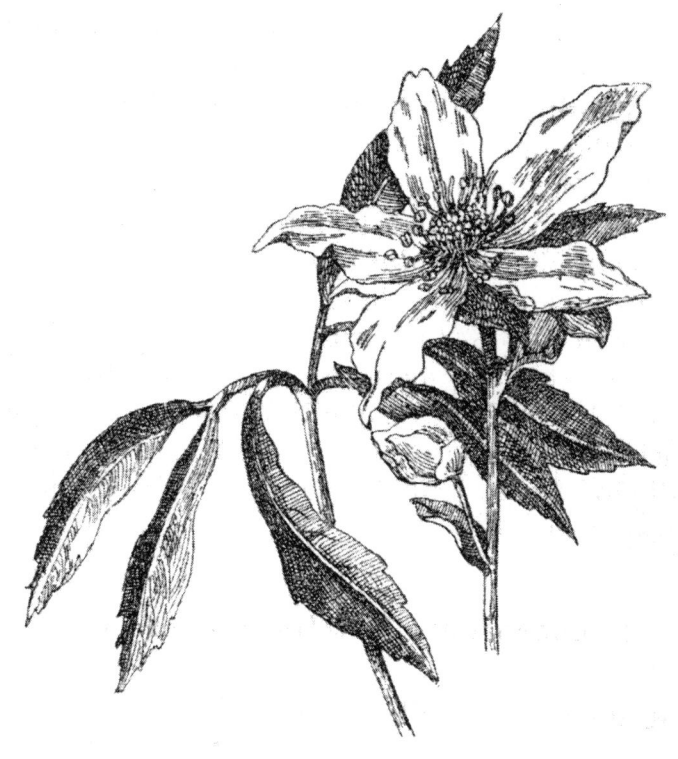

Squill (*Scilla maritima*, L.)

È una pianta che appartiene alla famiglia delle gigliacee; This plant belongs to the Liliaceae family; it grows on the sandy shores of the Mediterranean; it flowers in August. It has an ovoid bulb, the size of two fists, internally composed of fleshy tunics that are red or white, externally covered with thin dark brown membranes. The leaves are radical, smooth, glossy, dark green, oval, lanceolate, somewhat undulating. The stem is upright, simple, ranging from 65 centimeters to 1 meter in height, covered in its upper half with pedunculated, white flowers forming a long terminal spike; the fruit is a three-chambered capsule. The bulb is the only part of the plant used and contains an active substance, scillitin, which is non-crystallizable, soluble in alcohol, and has an acrid and very bitter taste.

In addition to the symptoms of intense gastroenteritis, squill produces a violent inflammation of the kidneys. Death usually occurs with delirium, convulsions, pupillary miosis, and other symptoms of irritation of the nerve centers (*Cantari*).

Treatment includes tannin; opiates, soothing and mucilaginous drinks; symptomatic care.

Ipecac (*Cephælis ipecacuanha*).

It is a small shrub that grows in the dense and shady forests of Brazil. The roots of this Rubiaceae are fibrous or represent a kind of elongated tubercles with very close annular grooves; they are almost woody and irregularly branched, with a brown epidermis under which lies a white parenchyma, fleshy when fresh; their center is occupied by a woody, filiform axis.

The stem, which is initially underground, straightens up and rises to about 35 centimeters; it is simple, quadrangular, somewhat hairy at the upper part. The leaves, numbering 6-8, are opposite, oval, acuminate, 5-10 centimeters long. The small, white flowers form a terminal panicle.

From the bark of the roots of this plant, an active principle, emetine ($C_{30}H_{40}N_2O_5$), an alkaloid that appears as an amorphous, white or yellowish powder with a bitter taste, was first isolated by *Pelletier* and *Magendie*. It is slightly soluble in cold water, very soluble in alcohol and ether, and forms crystallizable salts with acids. It is a very potent poison; ten to twenty centigrams are a lethal dose for a dog; a similar dose already causes violent vomiting in humans.

Symptoms of poisoning. - The ingestion of toxic doses of ipecac or its alkaloid is promptly followed by copious, repeated, and persistent vomiting, intense colic pain, and profuse diarrhea, prostration, depression, and, in more severe cases, a drop in temperature, collapse, and death due to cardiac paralysis.

Treatment. - Tannic acid, black coffee. Symptomatic care (stimulants, etc.)

BLOOD POISONS

The toxic substances of this group, upon entering the organism, exert a special action on oxyhemoglobin, causing chemical modifications that prevent hematosis..

Potassium Chlorate (KClO^3).

Potassium chlorate crystallizes in anhydrous, transparent, rhomboidal plates; it is insoluble in alcohol, soluble in water. It is widely used in laboratories to prepare oxygen and as an oxidizing agent; it is employed in pyrotechnics and in the manufacture of gunpowder, in textile printing, and in many other industries.

The lethal dose for adults is calculated at less than 15 grams; *Osborne* charged this salt with producing cerebral congestion and convulsions in children even at minimum doses (25 or 50 centigrams). *Abramans* saw a three-year-old child die from uremic symptoms after nine hours, following the ingestion of two grams of this salt. Absorption is very rapid; indeed, after five minutes, potassium chlorate can be found in the urine and saliva.

Poisonings mostly occur following the ingestion of a large

dose of potassium chlorate, often on an empty stomach and instead of magnesium sulfate.

Symptoms of poisoning. - Sharp pain in the gastric region, violent diarrhea with meteorism, persistent vomiting, dyspnea, cyanosis, and cardiac weakness, oliguria with urine typically being dark-greenish or reddish, containing a lot of albumin; hematin and methemoglobin are present. Furthermore, uremic phenomena are noted: delirium, exhaustion, tonic and clonic convulsions, followed by deep collapse and death within a few hours.

Anatomical lesions. - Parenchymatous inflammation of the heart, liver, gastric mucosa, and kidneys; the renal tubules are shown to be obstructed by pigmented masses. The blood is chocolate-colored; spectroscopic examination reveals the characteristic band of methemoglobin; microscopic examination shows considerable leukocytosis, poikilocytosis, and a reduction in the solid constituents of the blood.

Treatment. - Prophylaxis consists of never administering large doses of potassium chlorate on an empty stomach; it is better to give small doses on a full stomach, and take special care in febrile conditions and in diseases of the heart and lungs.

Treatment consists of gastric lavage and the administration of sodium bicarbonate orally and via enemas. Subsequently, cardiac stimulants (alcohol, camphor, caffeine, etc.), purgatives, diuretics, and diaphoretics (hot baths, pilocarpine, etc.) are resorted to.

Carbon Monoxide (CO).

It is a permanent, colorless, tasteless, and odorless gas that develops from the combustion of coal in an insufficient amount of air (poorly ventilated stoves, red-hot cast iron stoves, heaters of imperfect construction, combustion in enclosed spaces), in mine tunnels where explosions of gunpowder or guncotton are frequent. Carbon monoxide is much more dangerous and active than carbon dioxide; in fact, a ratio of 0.1:100 of this gas is enough to make the air unbreathable.

Symptoms. - They are very similar to those produced by carbon dioxide: severe headache, nausea, extreme prostration, inability to move or call for help, loss of consciousness, delirium, death.

The anatomical lesions found are identical to those of carbon dioxide asphyxiation; the treatment is the same.

Carbon Disulfide
(*Sulfocarbonic Anhydride,* $C S^2$).

Carbon disulfide, prepared by passing sulfur vapors through burning coal, is a clear, colorless liquid with an acrid, burning taste and a fetid, penetrating odor. It is highly volatile, insoluble in water, soluble in alcohol and ether, and extremely flammable; it burns with a dim flame in the air, producing carbon dioxide and sulfur dioxide; it dissolves sulfur, phosphorus, iodine, bromine, resins, rubber, fats, etc. It is used to degrease wool, in the extraction of oils and many aromatic substances, in galvanic silvering, to vulcanize and dissolve rubber, and to combat phylloxera.

Poisoning by inhalation of these harmful gases is generally observed in workers at rubber manufacturing plants; the resulting disorders are very persistent and can also cause death.

Symptoms. - Intoxication is primarily manifested by anemia, general thinness and weakness, loss of appetite, vomiting, involuntary emission of urine with a sulfur odor, and especially with serious nervous disorders: memory loss, decreased visual capacity, anesthesia, tremors, convulsions, and paralysis. Several of the patients observed by *Delpech* became insane.

Anatomical lesions. - These are mainly found in the blood, which is black due to numerous masses of pigment and the resultant destruction of red blood cells.

Symptomatic **treatment**.

Hydrogen Sulfide ($H_2 S$).

Hydrogen sulfide, also known as hydrosulfuric acid, is gaseous at room temperature. It is decomposed by chlorine, bromine, and iodine, with the deposition of sulfur and formation of a hydrogenated compound of the employed metalloid. It has a very unpleasant and penetrating odor of rotten eggs and is highly toxic when inhaled, but large quantities of its solution in water (sulfurous waters) can be consumed without danger. Hydrogen sulfide causes instant death when inhaled in its pure form; accidental poisonings are usually caused by emissions from sewers and latrines, manure heaps, etc.; sometimes they have been observed from sulfurous baths.

This gas is very easily absorbed by the lung mucosa and combines with the blood's hemoglobin to form sulfhemoglobin, which cannot sustain life.

Symptoms of poisoning. - In mild cases, when the breathed air is only slightly contaminated with the gas, headache, nausea, vomiting, abdominal pain, and diarrhea are observed. In more severe cases, a sense of heaviness in the stomach and temples is quickly followed by loss of consciousness, dyspnea, cyanosis, convulsions, paralysis, death.

Anatomical lesions. - Extremely foul odor of all organs and body cavities; lungs, liver, and other internal organs engorged with dark, fluid blood.

Treatment. - Prevention involves ventilating the area well or creating active combustion.

The poisoned individual should immediately be taken to fresh air, cautiously inhaling chlorine gas (chlorine water) if necessary, and artificial respiration should be performed, and in the most serious cases, blood transfusion. Emetics (apomorphine) may also be beneficial; the clothing of the poisoned should be treated with chlorine.

Pyrogallic acid (C^{6}H^3 [OH]^3)

This acid crystallizes into needles or plates of a brilliant white, odorless, with an extremely bitter and astringent taste, highly soluble in water. It is used in photography and forms the base of many hair dyes. It possesses very strong toxic properties; a solution of 2-4 grams is a lethal dose.

According to *Personne,* the symptomatology of poisoning is similar to that observed in phosphorus poisoning; pyrogallic acid also removes oxygen from the blood, causing more or less rapid asphyxiation.

The urine and vomited substances are black.

The observation of a 23-year-old man who swallowed 15 grams of pyrogallic acid diluted in a glass of water with added absinthe is reported by *Dalché.* He immediately felt a burning sensation in the esophagus and stomach, with severe and repeated black vomiting, increased temperature, black and albuminous urine, muscle cramps and soreness, leading to death in a coma after three days. Autopsy revealed no lesions in the digestive tract.

The lungs, heart, and brain were healthy. The kidneys were somewhat enlarged and blackish; the renal tubules were filled with refractive spheres that were not formed elements; there were clots in the capillaries and large veins. All the various lesions found indicated a profound alteration of the blood.

Even the application of pyrogallic acid on the skin is not without dangers; *Dollonar* observed the development of toxic nephritis in a 60-year-old man following the application of a 10:100 pyrogallol ointment to treat common psoriasis.

Treatment. - Mustard plasters on the chest and legs; alcohol, hypodermic injections of ether. Oxygen inhalations, artificial respiration.

Printed in Great Britain
by Amazon